Victorian Hernia Cures

LOCHLAINN SEABROOK WRITES IN THE FOLLOWING GENRES

Adult
Alternate History
American Civil War
American History
American Politics
American South
Ancient History
Anthropology
Apocrypha
Aviation
Biblical Exegesis
Biblical Hermeneutics
Biography
Children
Christian Mysticism
Coffee Table
Comparative Mythology
Comparative Religion
Cooking
Cryptozoology
Diet and Nutrition
Education
Encyclopediology
Entertainment
Ethnic Studies
Etymology
European History
Evolutionary Biology
Exposés
Family Histories
Film
Genealogy
Ghost Stories
Gospels
Health and Fitness
Historical Fiction
Historical Nonfiction
History
Humanities
Humor
Illustrations
Law of Attraction
Lexicography
Life After Death

Matriarchy
Men
Metaphysics
Military History
Mysteries and Enigmas
Mysticism
Natural Health
Natural History
Onomastics
Paleography
Paleontology
Paranormal
Patriarchy
Philosophy
Photography
Pictorial
Poetry
Politics
Prehistory
Presidential History
Quiz
Reference
Religion
Revolutionary Period
Science
Scripture
Self-help
Social Sciences
Spirituality
Spiritualism
Sport Science
Technology
Thanatology
Thealogy
Theology
UFOlogy
Vexillology
Victorian Period
War
Western
Wildlife
Women
World History
Young Adult

Mr. Seabrook does not author books for fame and glory, but for the love of writing and sharing his knowledge.

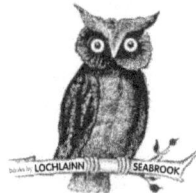

Be curious, not judgmental.

SeaRavenPress.com

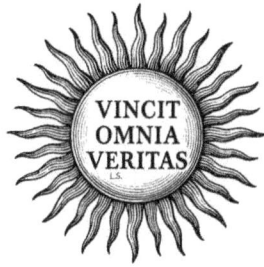

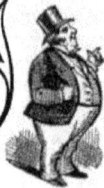

Warning: SEA RAVEN PRESS BOOKS WILL EXPAND YOUR ★ MIND!

VICTORIAN
HERNIA CURES

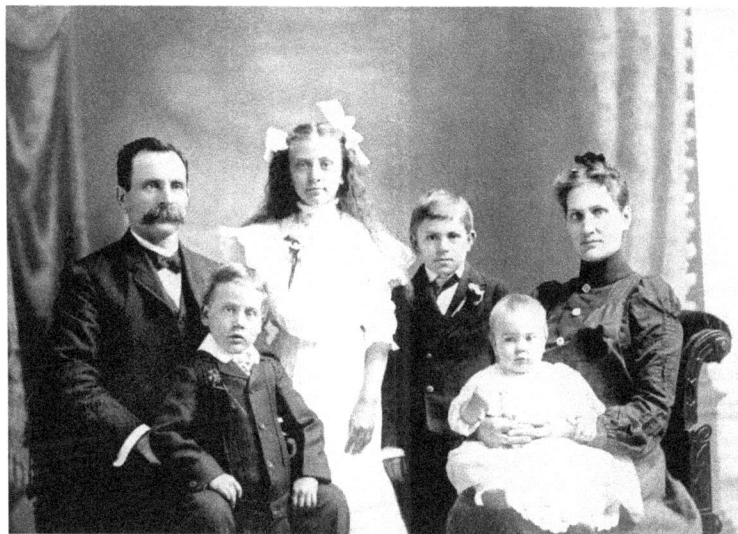

Nonsurgical Self-Treatment of Inguinal Hernia

LOCHLAINN SEABROOK
JEFFERSON DAVIS HISTORICAL GOLD MEDAL WINNER

Diligently Researched and Generously Illustrated
by the Author for the Elucidation of the Reader

2022

Sea Raven Press, Nashville, Tennessee, USA

VICTORIAN HERNIA CURES

Published by
Sea Raven Press, LLC, founded 1995
Nashville, Tennessee, USA
SeaRavenPress.com

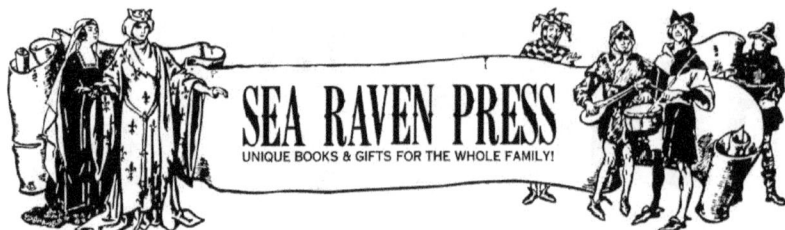

SEA RAVEN PRESS
UNIQUE BOOKS & GIFTS FOR THE WHOLE FAMILY!

PRINTING HISTORY
1st SRP paperback edition, 1st printing, April 2022. Updated August 2024 • ISBN: 978-1-955351-16-4
1st SRP hardcover edition, 1st printing, April 2022. Updated August 2024 • ISBN: 978-1-955351-17-1

ISBN: 978-1-955351-16-4 (paperback)
Library of Congress Control Number: 2022935611

Victorian Hernia Cures: Nonsurgical Self-Treatment of Inguinal Hernia, by Lochlainn Seabrook. Includes an introduction, illustrations, index, endnotes, appendices, and bibliography.

ARTWORK
Front and back cover design and art, book design, layout, font selection, and interior art by Lochlainn Seabrook
All images, image captions, graphic design, and graphic art copyright © Lochlainn Seabrook
All images selected, placed, manipulated, cleaned, colored, tinted, and/or created by Lochlainn Seabrook
Cover image: "Exercise is Key," Lochlainn Seabrook © copyright

All persons who approve of the authority and principles of Colonel Lochlainn Seabrook's literary work, and realize its benefits as a means of reeducating the world about facts left out of mainstream books, are hereby requested to avidly recommend his titles to others and to vigorously cooperate in extending their reach, scope, and influence around the globe.

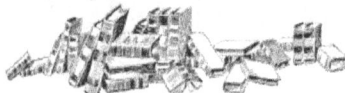

The alternative health and complimentary medical views expressed in this book are those of the publisher.

WRITTEN, DESIGNED, PUBLISHED, PRINTED, & MANUFACTURED IN THE UNITED STATES OF AMERICA

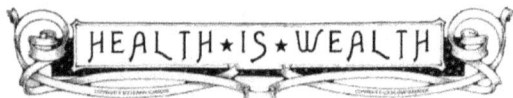

HEALTH ★ IS ★ WEALTH

DEDICATION

To the courageous Victorian men and women who disregarded the myopic pronouncements of the medical establishment, and endured slander and ridicule, in an effort to bring comfort and healing to the world's millions of hernia sufferers. We are your grateful patrons.

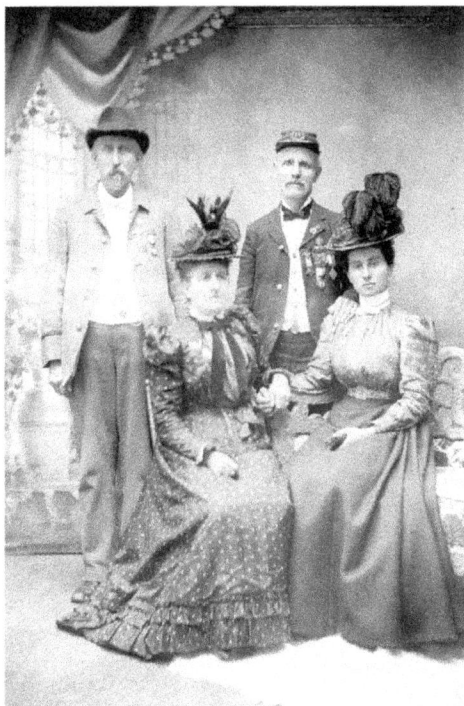

EPIGRAPH

Hernia, certainly intentionally, systematically, and frequently cured, the [former belief] that it was incurable, becomes futile . . . for cure, by intentional means, has been discovered . . . a newly discovered treatment . . . [that is] applicable to ruptures in their worst state, of adults of both sexes and of all ages.

Dr. William Dufour, 1821
SURGEON TO THE INSTITUTION FOR THE RADICAL CURE OF RUPTURE & OF STRICTURE
London, United Kingdom

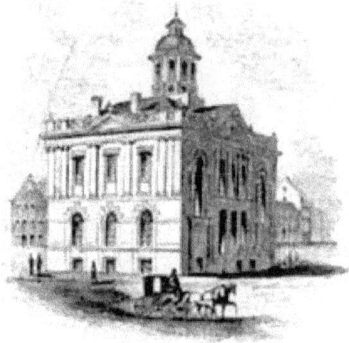

CONTENTS

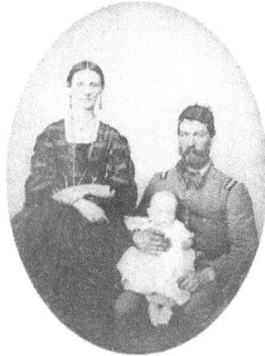

CHAPTER ONE

Victorian Descriptions of Hernial Anatomy

CHAPTER TWO

VICTORIAN EXPLANATIONS OF CAUSES OF INGUINAL HERNIA

CHAPTER THREE

VICTORIAN HOME TREATMENTS FOR INGUINAL HERNIA

CHAPTER FOUR
SEABROOK'S MODERN HERNIA SELF-TREATMENT PROGRAM

SRP

DISCLAIMER

❦ The contents of this book are for educational, informational, and historical purposes only and may not be construed as medical advice.

❦ The contents of this book are not a substitute for advice from a licensed healthcare provider, and are not intended to replace the services of a physician. Neither do they constitute a doctor-patient relationship.

❦ You should not rely solely on the contents of this book.

❦ You should not use the information in this book for diagnosing, treating, curing, or preventing a disease or any other medical health condition.

❦ Always consult a physician in all matters relating to your health, and particularly in respect to any symptoms that may require diagnosis or medical attention.

❦ Any action on your part in response to the information provided in this book is at your own risk and discretion.

❦ Neither the publisher or the author assume any obligation or liability—and make no warranties—with respect to the information provided in this book, including what may be obsolete data, inaccuracies, contradictions, spelling errors, etc. It is your responsibility to determine the value of this book's content.

❦ Owning, possessing, borrowing, reading, or using this book or its contents in any manner whatsoever infers that you have read, understand, and agree to this Disclaimer and all of the terms and conditions contained therein—without exception.

THE PUBLISHER

NOTES TO THE READER

DIFFERENTIATING THE AUTHOR FROM THE CONTRIBUTORS
❶ Throughout this book my writing (the author) is in normal text (example). The writings of contributors are always in **bold text** and are, in most cases, preceded by a Victorian hand pointer (☛).

A WORD ON VICTORIAN MATERIAL
❷ In order to preserve the authentic historicity of the past, I have retained the original spellings, formatting, and punctuation of the Victorians I quote. These include such items as Old European and British-English spellings, long-running paragraphs, obsolete words, and various literary devices peculiar to the time. Bracketed words within quotes are my additions and clarifications, while italicized words within quotes are (where indicated) my emphasis.

VICTORIAN PERIOD
❸ Though some of the medical professionals cited in this book wrote after the Victorian Era ended in 1901, all were born during the Victorian Era (which began in 1837), and so are considered Victorians.

CONTENT WARNING
❹ Some of the material in this book may not be suitable for children. Parental guidance is suggested.

FURTHER YOUR EDUCATION
❺ For those interested in further educating themselves on the topics of alternative health and self-healing, please see my "Mind, Body, Spirit" books—listed in the Bibliography.

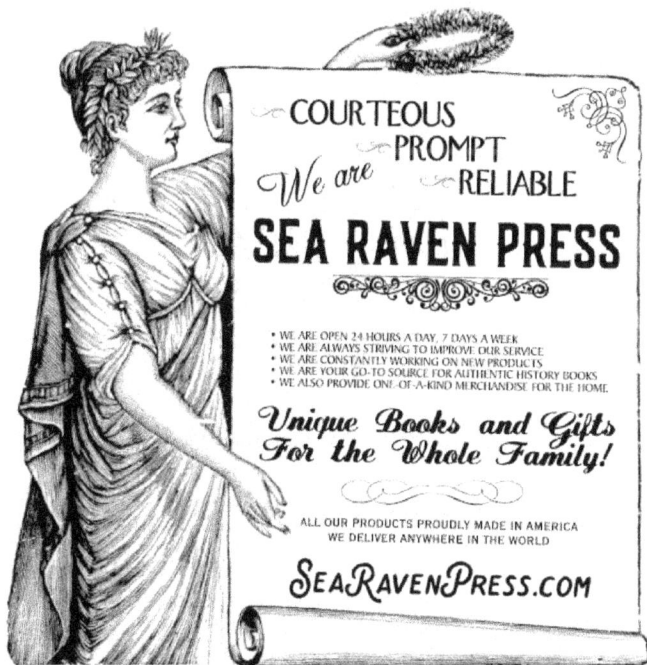

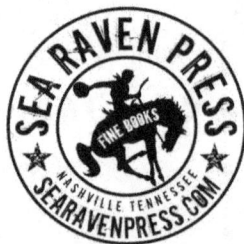

INTRODUCTION

"From circumstances which have come to my knowledge, I think it possible that something more than is yet generally known may be done for persons afflicted with hernia."

Sir William Fergusson, 1ˢᵗ Baronet
CHAIR OF SURGERY, KING'S COLLEGE, LONDON, UK, 1870

IS THIS BOOK FOR YOU?

ACCORDING TO 19ᵀᴴ-CENTURY STATISTICS, ONE in seven men and one in 12 women will acquire a hernia,[1] and most of these will be inguinal hernias,[2] the most common type of at least 20 or more varieties that were then recognized.[3] In 1893, out of a total population of 63 million people, it was estimated that at least 4 million Americans, or about 6.3 percent, were suffering from a hernia of one kind or another.[4]

Early 20ᵗʰ-Century physician Dr. A. D. Bevan of Presbyterian Hospital in Chicago, Illinois, reported that in 1916,

☛ **. . . hernia occurs in about 12 percent of the males and in about 2 percent of the females, that is, about one man out of eight some time in his life has a rupture, and about one woman out of fifty.[5]**

Noted Victorian physician Dr. Charles A. Lauffer remarked that when it comes to the working class alone,

☛ **. . . hernia occurs with sufficient frequency to be regarded as the greatest single frailty of the American worker. The . . . inguinal type comprises over 92 percent of all hernias encountered.[6]**

If you have an inguinal hernia yourself, you are far from alone. In 1926, the U.S. Navy reported that out of 434 cases of hernia, surgical operations were performed on:

403 inguinal hernias.
15 ventral hernias.
6 hernias of muscle.
4 epigastric hernia.

3 femoral hernia.
3 umbilical hernia.[7]

In 1984, some 469,000 repairs of inguinal hernia were performed across the U.S.[8] According to the FDA, today (2022) "more than one million hernia repairs are performed each year in the U.S.," and of these approximately 800,000 are to repair inguinal hernias.[9]

SOME REQUIREMENTS FOR SELF-TREATMENT

Note that the above figures disregard the many tens of thousands of individuals who, for one reason or another, do not seek, need, or want medical surgery for their inguinal hernia. If you are one of these men or women, this book is for you.

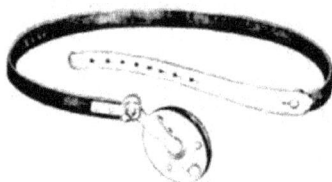

Victorian adjustable ball-and-socket hernia belt, known then as a truss.

However, this is not the only qualification.

• It will also be helpful if you are a determined, disciplined, self-motivated adult who is willing to work hard, make sacrifices, and delay gratification, always keeping the end goal in mind through the inevitable ups and downs that come with home treatment.

• You should be first examined by a doctor to make sure that your particular inguinal hernia type (note that there are different forms, some extremely dangerous) and location, as well as your overall health condition, permit hernia self-treatment.

• Your inguinal hernia should *not* be the result of a violent trauma to the body (known as a traumatic hernia); that is, a hernia caused by an injury. For this would normally result in an actual tear (i.e., an *artificial* hole) in the abdominal tissues. While this type of hernia is quite rare,[10] it not only lacks the preformed hernial sac of a true hernia,[11] it is among those types most likely to require surgery. To qualify then, your hernia should be diagnosed as a congenital hernia. The congenital or hereditary hernia seems to produce weak abdominal muscles in the fetal stages, which later in life spontaneously result in the protrusion of viscera through a *normal* but flaccid opening in the tissues of the abdomen. It is this type of inguinal hernia, the congenital inguinal hernia, that seems most conducive to home self-treatment.[12] (After diagnosis, your doctor can advise you properly on this question.)

• Lastly, and perhaps most importantly, your inguinal hernia must be reducible. That is, if and when it "pops" out, you must be able to manually push the protrusion back into place behind your abdominal wall.[13]

If you meet all of these requirements, I believe you will find the information in the following pages of both great interest and great help in possibly resolving your hernia issues.

TWO SCHOOLS OF THOUGHT
The medical world is divided into two opposing and highly acrimonious camps regarding reducible inguinal hernia: those who believe that it cannot heal on its own and therefore always requires surgery, and those who maintain that it can and will heal on its own and therefore seldom if ever requires surgery (this second group believes the scalpel to be an absolute hindrance to healing a hernia). I will refer to the former group as the *Conventional School of Medicine* and the latter as the *Natural School of Medicine*.

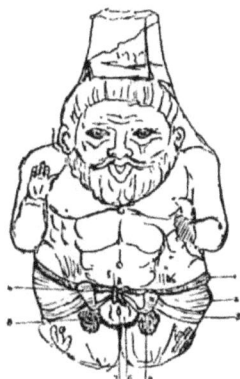

The question immediately arises: which school is correct?

Due to the infinite physical and mental differences in each individual hernia sufferer, the answer is not black and white. In fact, for some, surgery would be the right decision, while for others nonsurgical self-treatment would be the course to choose. Thus, this question can and must only be answered by you and by your doctor.

Inguinal hernias are as old as humanity. The artist who sculpted this 3,000 year old statue of the Egyptian god Bes (discovered in an ancient Phoenician cemetery), portrayed the deity wearing a truss for a double inguinal hernia.

However, having said this, there are a number of factors that point to the superiority of using natural non-medical methods to cure inguinal hernias—the very subject of this book.

As I will show in the following pages, the *first cause* or *main cause* of nearly all inguinal hernias is not from an external trauma to the body (such as heavy lifting). That would be a *secondary* or "*exciting cause*," as Victorian doctors called it. The actual first cause, as alluded to above, is genetic inheritance, which, in the case of inguinal hernias, bestows upon one weak abdominal musculature. Hence, this type of hernia is called a *congenital hernia* (because the conditions it produces are formed in utero).

Congenital hernias provide an ideal environment for the secondary or exciting cause, which is what actually prompts an organ to push through either the individual's innate flabby abdominal wall or a natural but abnormally wide hole in the abdominal tissue, both which would be lacking in an individual who did not have this condition. This, the exciting cause, could be almost anything, from jumping and coughing to sneezing and falling, and yes, heavy lifting.

A congenital hernia differs greatly from its primary counterpart, the *traumatic hernia*, whose main cause is the secondary, immediate, or exciting cause in congenital hernias; namely, violent exertion. Thus traumatic hernia is the direct result of, not weak abdominal muscles, as in congenital hernias, but rather a usually sudden and severe trauma to the body. The important fact to note here is that this often results in a literal tear in the abdominal tissues, which then allows the viscera to protrude. Despite this, the traumatic hernia does not have a hernial sac, which is a sign of a true hernia.[14]

It is apparent from this that a traumatic hernia not only differs from a congenital hernia in its main cause, it also differs in its secondary cause, its structure, and what kind of treatment it requires. And this is good news for those suffering from this specific affliction.

Why?

WHY CONGENITAL HERNIA IS USUALLY SELF-TREATABLE
A reducible inguinal hernia, which is what most of my readers will have, is, in almost every case, an *inborn disease*, while a traumatic hernia is an *injury*. In simple terms, a disease is more amenable to self-treatment than a serious injury, which almost always requires medical treatment—in the case of hernias, usually surgery.

The Natural School of Medicine, whose main focus has always been something that utilizes the body's own amazing curative powers, naturally turns to self-treatment for reducible inguinal hernia. By the same token, it rejects medical interference, such as surgery, considering it a deterrent to healing. The Conventional School, on the other hand, focuses on what it knows, which is medications and surgery, rejecting anything "natural" as dangerous pseudoscience.

Why most of today's conventional doctors and surgeons refuse to consider self-treatment for inguinal hernia is a question best put to them. They certainly have never tried to hide their animus toward natural hernia treatments, as can be seen in the following statement made in 1918 by Dr. Carl Goodwin Burdick and Dr.

Bradley L. Coley. Believing (incorrectly) that hernia belt makers are disreputable companies only interested in profit, and that there is no "permanent cure" for hernias except surgery, they made this caustic remark:

☞ . . . until the laity has been educated not to believe the exaggerated claims made by the vast majority of truss makers, many will still cling to this form of treatment.[15]

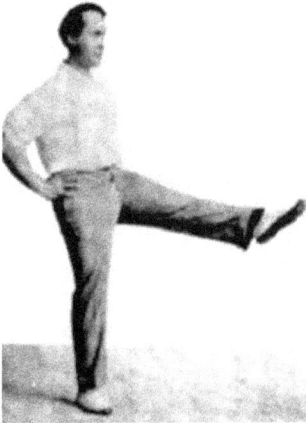

As we shall see, according to many Victorian doctors, physical fitness work outs—particularly those that strengthen the abdominal muscles—are a vital component in the self-treatment of reducible inguinal hernia.

This empirical and arrogant attitude, long well-known among establishment doctors, has a long history. Attentive school students will remember that

☞ it was the [conventional] medical profession that drove [noted German physician Franz Anton] Mesmer into a dishonored exile and a premature grave for the sole reason that he healed the sick without the use of pills. [Not only that, they] ridiculed, proscribed, and ostracized every medical man who dared conduct an honest investigation of mesmeric phenomena.[16]

EMBRACING THE NATURAL SCHOOL OF MEDICINE
Admittedly, my description of the two medical schools of thought is somewhat over simplistic, for, though rare, there are some conventional doctors who are open to the natural view, while there are some natural doctors who are open to the conventional view. Nonetheless, my research and experience has shown that my categorization of the two schools is basically accurate.

Obviously, *Victorian Hernia Cures* embraces the teachings of the Natural School of Medicine, for the very purpose of this book is to resuscitate centuries-old information on self-healing of reducible inguinal hernia; beneficial medical information that was familiar and well established in the 19th Century, but much of which today has been lost, forgotten, or intentionally suppressed.

WHY I WROTE THIS BOOK

I have been heavily immersed in the fields of health, fitness, and nutrition for many decades, and once helped found and operate a natural foods store. This does not make me a doctor, of course; nor even an authority in these areas—and I make no pretensions as such.

Yet, after years of study and self-experimentation, I have accrued a great deal of knowledge about the body-mind-spirit complex that is no longer taught in modern medical schools, but which was common and accepted by doctors before 1900. I put this old time wisdom to good use by healing myself of many ailments, such as cancer, dental disease, and cluster headaches, all without the "aid" of doctors, pills, or scalpels. It is obvious that there are things modern mainstream medicine does not know, for it claims that all of the illnesses I was able to rid myself of have no known cure.

Dissection of an internal or direct inguinal hernia.

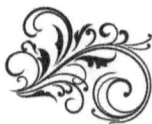

Thus, when it came time to find "Nature's cure" for my inguinal hernia, I automatically turned to the past, which as a neo-Victorian writer, researcher, and historian, meant perusing my old dusty collection of 19th-Century books. It was here, after years of pouring over thousands of faded and torn pages, that I discovered the natural hernia cure I was looking for. And though it thoroughly violates the beliefs of the Conventional School of Medicine, I can testify that it works, for I used it to successfully treat and eliminate my inguinal hernia in a matter of just a few months.

While I devote the first three chapters of *Victorian Hernia Cures* to the engrossing findings and opinions of 19th- and early 20th-Century hernia doctors, the fourth and final chapter contains a condensation of the first three chapters, along with my own discoveries and views. This material I have reformulated and written out as a modern guide, complete with anatomical information, instructional details, and muscle building exercises.

If this little book helps one individual take control of his or her own hernia health, I will have accomplished my goal.

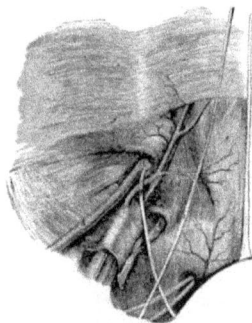

Lochlainn Seabrook
Nashville, Tennessee, USA
April 2022

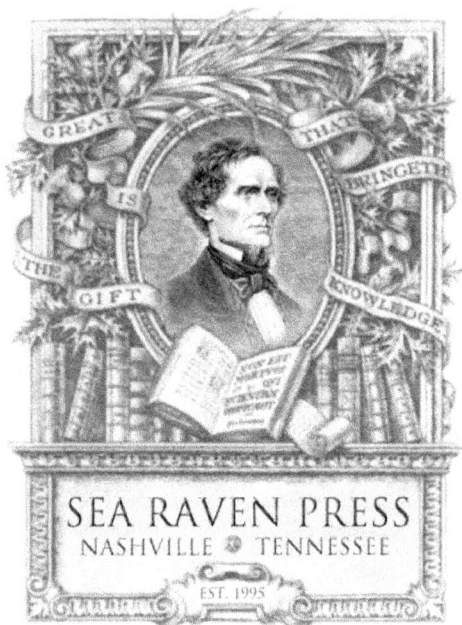

SEA RAVEN PRESS
NASHVILLE ❀ TENNESSEE
EST. 1995

"Books invite all; they constrain none."
Hartley Burr Alexander (1873-1939)

CHART OF THE INGUINAL REGION
showing its tissues, parts, and organs on front of torso

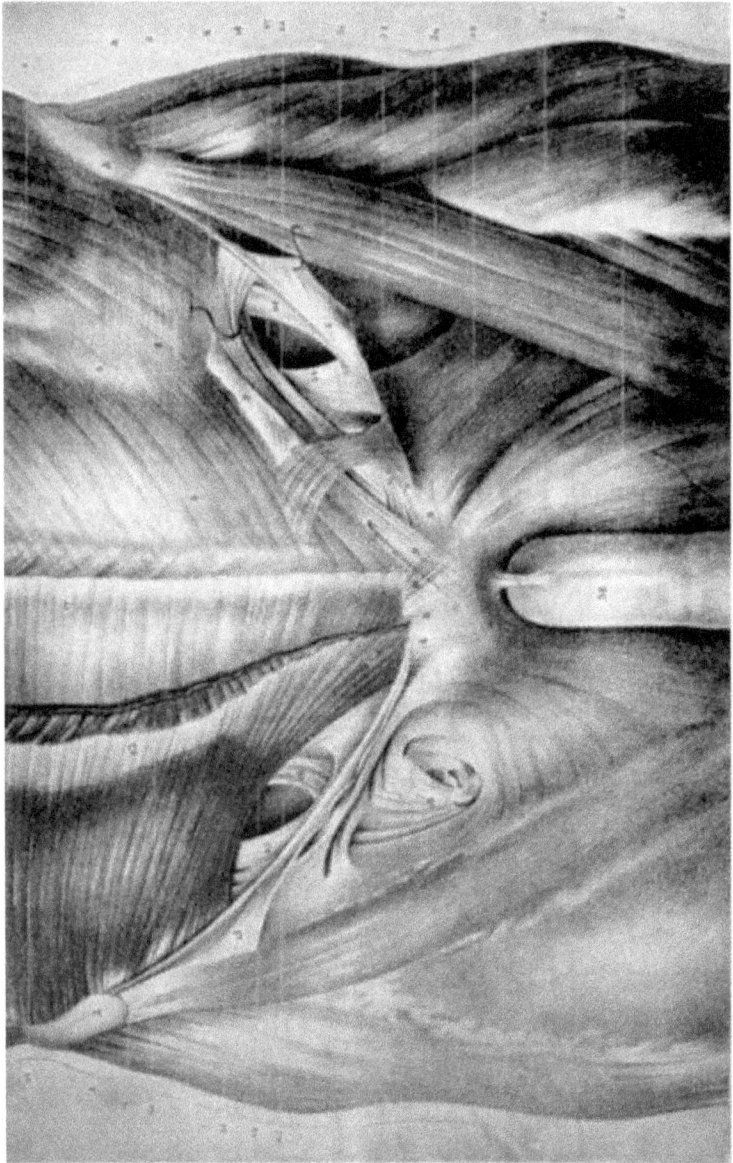

(To study the chart above, rotate book to the right. See following two pages for description.)

Study of the Inguinal Canal

By Jean-Baptiste Marc Bourgery (1797-1849)

FROM THE BOOK *A PRACTICAL TREATISE ON HERNIA*,
BY JOSEPH H. WARREN, 1880

(As a curiosity of language, the description of the chart on the foregoing page will be given in the words of the original French translation. J. H. W.)

Details of the inferior extremity of the Great Oblique and Transversal, and their relations with the Groins and origin of the Thighs.

———⚬✦❧❀✦———

Left side of the Subject: Great oblique, whose aponeurosis is half open, and thrown back to shew the interior of the inguinal canal, the cremaster being removed. The circumference of the ring is preserved in [the] form of a stay. The thigh represents the upper extremity of the superficial muscles.

Right side: Femoral transversal and aponeurosis.

EXPLANATION OF THE CHART

A, A. Anterior and superior iliac spines.

B, B. Pubic spines.

LEFT SIDE

1. Inferior extremity of the great oblique.
2, 2. Its aponeurosis.
3, 3. Shreds of the aponeurosis, inverted, to show the inguinal canal.
5. Origin of [François] Poupart's ligament.
6. Cut of the small bands, from whence the external pillar proceeds.
7. External pillar, implanted upon the spine of the pubis.
8. Small band, from whence the internal pillar proceeds.
9. Internal pillar. Between the two pillars is the inguinal ring.
10. Internal inguinal ligament.
11. Extremity of the internal pillar of the right side.
12. First band of insertion to the pubis, separated from the internal pillar by the arcade of passage to the ilio-scrotal nerve.
13. Extremity of the aponeurosis which closes the ring, preserved in form of a stay.

RIGHT SIDE

14. Origin of Poupart's ligament in the iliac spinal.
15. *Aponeurosis*, thrown back upon the thigh.
16. Its tie, forming the external pillar.
17. Aponeurosis of the little oblique, in front of the great right.
18. *Left side:* Last ties of this muscle in the gutter of Poupart's ligament. The arcade which it forms is raised up by a hook, to let the transversal be seen.
19. *Right side:* Extremity of the fibres of the little oblique inverted within, to let the aponeurosis of the transversal be seen.
20. Idem. Transversal.
21. Idem. Last ties of this muscle in the gutter of Poupart's ligament.
22, 22. Summit of the arcade which it forms above the internal orifice of the inguinal canal.
23. Aponeurosis of the transversal.
24. Inferior tie of the pubis. It is the same aponeurosis which is seen through the orifice of the left inguinal ring.
25, 25. *Of the sides:* Thick edge of the fascia-transversalis, which limits the superior orifice of the inguinal canal outside, and then unites itself with the gutter of Poupart's ligament.
26, 26. Idem. Very fine portion of the same fascia, which forms the internal edge of the orifice. Behind a fibro-cellulous sheet are seen the epigastric vessels which ascend parallelly to the internal edge.
26, 27. Idem. Ellipsoidal internal orifice of the inguinal canal.
28. *Right side:* Superficial aponeurotic leaf, applied upon the crural vessels.
29. Iilem. Section of the internal sapheneous vein, which crosses the femoral aponeurosis (inferior crural ring), in order to through itself into the femoral vein.
30. *Left side:* Sartor muscle.
31. Fascia-lata.
32. Reflected mass of the psoas and iliac.
33. Péctiné.
34. Anterior right.
35. First abductor.
36. Reproductive organs.[17]

"SHALL THE MIND BE STRONG THE BODY MUST LEND IT THE STRENGTH."

Daniel Gottlieb Moritz Schreber, 1899

1

VICTORIAN DESCRIPTIONS OF HERNIAL ANATOMY

THE CONFUSING REALM OF HERNIA SCIENCE

When discussing the topic of inguinal hernias, we are entering a domain of countless complexities, vague abstractions, and worldwide professional disagreement. Victorian doctors, as we shall see, were befuddled both by the intricacies of the abdominal contents and by their fellow surgeons' findings and descriptions of hernia types, hernia operations, and hernia nomenclature.

Unfortunately, not much has changed since the 19th Century. While some generalities are now universally accepted, there is still no meeting of the minds among doctors on the precise causes, symptoms, and characteristics of inguinal hernia, with no two agreeing on everything. Hernia doctors cannot even find common ground on the proper surgical procedure, as army officer Strother B. Marshall, of the U.S. Medical Corps, writes in 1960:

☛ There is [as of yet] **no unanimity of opinion as to the best type of operation to be used for the ordinary, run-of-the-mine, primary indirect inguinal hernia.**[18]

Dr. James Johnson wrote the following in an 1822 issue of *The Medico-Surgical Review, and Journal of Medical Science:*

☞ The anatomy of hernia has lately occupied the attention of the most eminent surgeons, as [Astley] Cooper, [Antonio] Scarpa, Hey, etc., yet, notwithstanding the labours of these, and many others high in the profession, it remains still one of the most puzzling and confused subjects to the surgical pupil. This has arisen, we are convinced, not so much from the complicated nature of the structure, as from the confusion of terms and the endless differences in the descriptions; there is such a jumble of tendons and ligaments, straight and crooked, and sheaths and fascias, and arches, with pillars and rings, that the pupil is perfectly confounded and lost amongst them. But this is not the worst of it, for we find many different names applied to the same part, or to its subdivisions; for instance, the femoral ligament, the falciform process of the fascia lata, and the sheath of the vessels, etc., are all names applied to the same structure. Were surgeons and anatomists, by common consent, to abandon such superfluity of terms, (for when a name, however absurd, is once bestowed, it is seldom forgotten, especially by those who talk about anatomy), a great deal of difficulty would be done away with.[19]

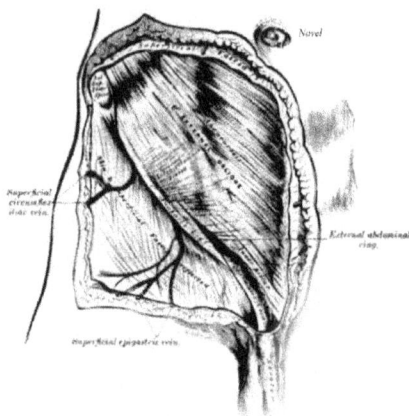

Inguinal hernia: A superficial dissection.

According to one "Mr. Lizars," a Victorian medical practitioner writing in the year 1832:

☞ Work after work has been published on the subject [of hernia], and the more and more confused and intricate are the descriptions. [Andreas] Vesalius, [Bartolomeo] Eustachius, [William] Cowper, [Bernhard S.] Albinus, Douglas, all have erred—and the anatomy of hernias may be pronounced the arcanum of surgery.[20]

Surely, if these intelligent and highly educated Victorian surgeons could not agree on what they referred to as the unknowable mysteries of hernias, we cannot expect to unravel their many enigmas in a small book of this nature.

While there are still many unanswered questions, as well as continuing debate over diagnosis and treatment, fortunately, there is much that is definitively known and much that we have learned about hernias since the 19ᵗʰ and early 20ᵗʰ Centuries. It is this knowledge that we will be exploring in this book.

BASIC ABDOMINAL ANATOMY
Any attempt at hernia self-healing must begin with a basic grasp of hernia science; and by this I mean a comprehension of the anatomy of the abdomen, and more specifically of the oblique fibers of the abdominal muscles where inguinal hernias form. Since we are following what I call the early Natural School of Medicine in this regard, we will be consulting the works and words of Victorian doctors—who we now turn to in order to deepen our understanding.

To begin with, let us familiarize ourselves with the relevant herniological definitions found in the 1916 work *The American Illustrated Medical Dictionary*, by W. A. Newman Dorland:

- *Hernia:* **The protrusion of a loop or knuckle of an organ tissue through an abnormal opening.**
- *Inguinal hernia:* **A hernia into the inguinal canal.**
- *Reducible hernia:* **One that may be returned by manipulation.**
- *Irreducible hernia:* **A hernia that cannot be restored by taxis** [from the Greek, meaning "the manual restoration of a displaced body part"].[21]
- *Congenital hernia:* **A hernia that exists at birth.** [Note: This is the most common type of hernia, and, as we shall discuss, was considered a curable "disease" during the 19ᵗʰ Century. Because it often forms slowly and almost imperceptibly—sometimes taking years or even decades to manifest—the "cause" of most congenital hernias is usually impossible to determine. Like "acquired hernia" (see below), this term is the cause of much bewilderment, as well as the subject of continued debate.[22] L.S.]
- *Acquired hernia:* **One brought on by lifting or by a strain or other injury.** [Note: Acquired hernias, which, according to to Victorian doctors, are actually quite rare (some say they are

nonexistent),[23] were considered an "injury" at the time, and were thus sometimes also referred to as "traumatic" or "accidental" hernias, depending on their initial exciting cause. Typically, acquired or traumatic hernias differ markedly from congenital hernias in that they lack a preformed hernial sac (the sign of a true hernia),[24] are of recent origin, appear suddenly, are accompanied by pain, and always immediately follow an accident.[25] For good reason, industrial companies maintain strict workers' compensation standards when it comes to defining an acquired or traumatic hernia: Besides the signs and symptoms above, **the injured man must have been forced to stop work immediately following the accident. He must have been forced to seek medical attention at once, or at most by the evening of the following day.**[26] Needless to say, much confusion also surrounds this term, as we shall see. L.S.]

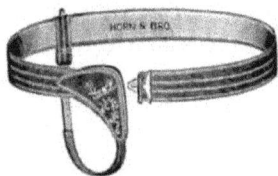

A Victorian elastic truss with special pad.

- *Direct inguinal hernia:* **One that passes directly through the abdominal wall by the internal ring.**
- *Ventral hernia:* **A hernia through the abdominal wall.**[27]

In his 1893 book *A Dictionary of Medical Science*, Dr. Robley J. Dunglison gives the following definitions:

- **Hernia: Any tumor formed by the displacement of a viscus, or a portion of a viscus which has escaped from its natural cavity by some aperture and projects externally. Herniae have been arranged according to the region or organs affected, the opening involved, or the viscera included in them.**
- **Abdominal herniae: are remarkable for their frequency, variety, and the danger attending them. They are produced by the protrusion of the viscera of the abdomen through the natural or accidental apertures in the parietes [the wall of an organ or bodily cavity] of that cavity. The organs forming them most frequently are the intestines and the epiploon. These herniae have been divided . . . according to the apertures by which they escape.**
- **Inguinal hernia: which issue by the inguinal canal, are called bubonocele when small, and scrotal hernia or**

oscheocele in man when they descend into the scrotum; or vulvar hernia or pudendal or labial hernia, episiocele, in women when they extend to the labia majora.[28]

In his 1908 book *Surgery*, the great Southern physician Dr. John Allan Wyeth writes:

☛ An inguinal hernia may be direct or indirect, complete or incomplete, congenital or acquired. The indirect or "oblique" variety is much more frequently met with. In the male, the contents pass into the internal abdominal ring, and follow the spermatic cord along the inguinal canal, at times descending into the tunica vaginalis testis. In the female, the descent is in the canal of Nuck, following the round ligament in the inguinal canal, and at times as far as the labium.[29]

In 1901 Dr. Henry Gray published his book *Anatomy, Descriptive and Surgical*, which contains the following definitions:

☛ Inguinal hernia is that form of protrusion which makes its way through the abdomen in the inguinal region. There are two principal varieties of inguinal hernia—external or oblique, and internal or direct.
    External or oblique inguinal hernia [also known as lateral],[30] the more frequent of the two, takes the same course as the spermatic cord. It is called external from the neck of the sac being on the outer or iliac side of the deep epigastric artery.
    Internal or direct inguinal hernia [also known as medial][31] does not follow the same course as the cord, but protrudes through the abdominal wall on the inner or pubic side of the deep epigastric artery.[32]

In his 1861 book *A Manual for the Practice of Surgery*, Thomas Bryant provides these descriptions of inguinal hernias:

☛ Inguinal hernia, or that form which protrudes through the internal or external abdominal rings, includes two-thirds of all cases of hernia, and about half of all cases of strangulated hernia. Two out of three cases of strangulated inguinal hernia are reducible by the taxis, the third requiring operation.

. . . An inguinal hernia is called *oblique* when it passes through the internal ring and along the inguinal canal downwards towards the scrotum; *direct*, when it does not pass through the internal ring, but through the external in a direct way.

The oblique, from being anatomically placed external to the deep epigastric artery, is called *external oblique*, while the direct from being internal to the same vessel is known as the *internal direct*.

When the oblique has not passed the external ring, it is known as a *bubonocele*; when the oblique or direct has passed into the scrotum it is called a *scrotal hernia* or *oscheocele*.

In the *oblique inguinal*, the sac of the hernia may be the natural vaginal process peritoneum that was formed on the descent of the testicle in fetal life, and has not closed, i.e., *a congenital sac*; or an *acquired sac* formed by the gradual pouching of the parietal peritoneum through the ring.

A schematic of the abdominal organs.

In the *direct inguinal*, the sac is always of the acquired form.[33]

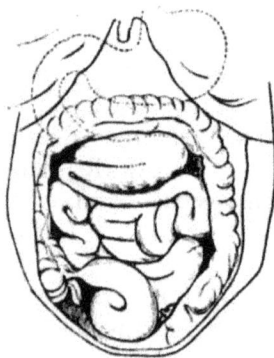

The following two herniary terms are germane to our discussion, both definitions which derive from the 1748 book *A Dissertation on Hernias or Ruptures*, by George M. Arnaud:

• *Complete hernia:* A hernia that descends into the scrotum in men, and into the labia pudendi in women.
• *Incomplete hernia:* A hernia that remains in the flexure [fold] of the groin.[34]

In his 1865 work *A Dictionary of Terms Used in Medicine and the Collateral Sciences*, Richard D. Hoblyn defines inguinal hernia this way:

• *Hernia inguinalis:* Bubonocele, or hernia at the groin; hernia which protrudes through one or both abdominal rings. It is termed *incomplete* or *oblique*, when it does not protrude directly through the external abdominal ring; and *complete* or *direct*, when it passes directly out at that opening.[35]

One other term is applicable. This definition is from Dr. Hermann Tillmanns' 1898 work *A Text-Book of Surgery*:

• *Hernial ring:* **The opening through which the hernia protrudes from the abdominal cavity. The opening in question may be either a normal or an abnormal one, arising, for example, from an injury. The different herniae are designated according to the location of this opening—e.g., inguinal hernia, femoral hernia, umbilical hernia, diaphragmatic hernia, etc.**[36]

Finally, we may divide the causes of inguinal hernias into two broad categories, a topic that will be covered in more detail in Chapter Two:

• *Main cause:* 1) The most common initial causative factor or principle cause (also sometimes known as predisposing cause) behind an inguinal hernia is *heredity*[37] (i.e., it is an inherited disease, one most well-known as a congenital hernia). 2) The second most common cause is an *injury* (i.e., a traumatic hernia—or acquired hernia, as it is also sometimes confusingly known).[38]
• *Exciting causes:* Defined by Victorian Dr. William B. Coley as: **"Anything which increases the intra-abdominal pressure may be the immediate exciting cause of a hernia. The most common of these causes are lifting, straining, and coughing."** Also known as immediate causes, other common exciting causes are falling [after losing one's balance], slipping, bronchitis, whooping-cough,[39] pregnancy, obesity, sneezing, direct blow to the abdomen, running, jumping, climbing,[40] overly vigorous coition,[41] and in men specifically, enlarged prostate.[42]

DEFINING & DESCRIBING HERNIAS
In his 1919 article "Hernia in Industry," industrial surgeon Dr. Charles A. Lauffer gives the following simple description of hernia:

☛ **A hernia is a protrusion, the essential part of which is** the hernial sac. The lining membrane of the body cavity is the peritoneum, and the hernial sac is a process of peritoneum shoved out from the body cavity, serving as a pocket for the reception of portions of omentum, intestine, or other abdominal organs.[43]

In 1916 Dr. Andrew A. Gour provides the following statements in his book *The Therapeutics of Activity*:

☛ The muscle fibres which form the pillars of the internal and external openings are fibres of the oblique and transversalis muscles. There are three layers of muscle: the inner layer is made up of the fibers of the transversalis muscle, the middle layer of the internal oblique, and the external layer of the external oblique muscle. The fibers of the external oblique pass downward from the lower six ribs, and the tendon is inserted at the anterior third of the crest of the ilium. At the pubic crest, between these two points, the muscle is folded upon itself in a tendinous structure that forms the basis of Poupart's ligament. At the lower third of the pubic spine the tendons of the transversalis and internal oblique muscles as well as that of the external, do not coalesce, but leave an arched opening called the external ring. There is a slit-like opening formed by a separation of the horizontal fibers of the transversalis, through which passes the spermatic cord in the male and the round ligament in the female. The passage from the internal to the external ring through which these structures pass, is called the inguinal canal. This canal is formed by the lack of coalescence of the fascia constituting the myolemma of the oblique muscles. It is an oblique canal about an inch and a half in length, directed downward and inward parallel with, and a little above, Poupart's ligament.

Into this canal, by way of the internal ring opening,

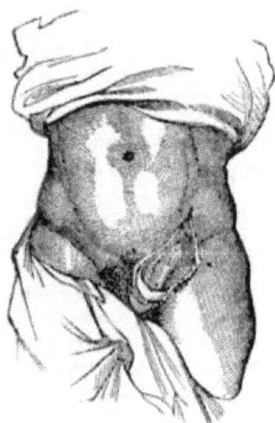

Dissection of the left inguinal region, showing the location of the external ring and the internal ring.

may pass any free viscus of suitable size. Once in the canal it may pass downward until it is checked at the super-pubic fascia or in the scrotum or vaginal labia. Not infrequently it distends the scrotum and produces a large swelling that hangs down several inches. This form of hernia is known as the indirect or oblique inguinal.

Where the protrusion penetrates some part of the abdominal wall internal to the epigastric artery it is called a direct inguinal, or internal oblique hernia. In this form the protrusion may escape from the abdomen through the fibers of the conjoined tendon or the tendon is gradually distended in front of it so as to form a complete investment for it.[44]

Dr. Gour goes on to impart the following detailed description of hernias:

☛ A hernia consists of the sac and its contents. The sac is made up of peritoneum and lining membrane of the abdominal cavity. The sac is divided into the mouth, the neck and body. The mouth is the aperture communicating with the abdominal cavity. The body is the expanded portion. The neck is the constricted part at the abdominal opening.

... The contents of the sac are omentum, intestine, or any movable contents of the abdomen. "In some cases," according to [William B.] De Garmo, "even a kidney or parts of the liver have been found in the hernial sac."

Herniae are divided clinically into the reducible, irreducible, incarcerated, inflamed and strangulated.

In *reducible inguinal hernia* the contents can be reduced into the abdominal cavity. The acquired sac is always reducible at first. That is, it is free from adhesions. Sooner or later adhesions are formed and render it permanent. The sac then forms a moist serous lining to the inguinal canal.

Irreducible hernia presents the usual symptoms of hernia, but cannot be replaced in the abdomen. A hernia that has been reducible may in time become irreducible because of adhesions, because of the growth of omental fat, or because of the increase in size of the mass. It may result in serious complications because of its prominence, which renders it liable to bruise and thus give pain, or there is always danger of obstruction and strangulation. Irreducible hernia usually requires surgery.

Incarcerated or obstructed means a condition in which there is an obstruction caused by the damming up of feces or undigested food. The fecal current is stopped but the blood flow in the intestinal walls is undisturbed. This condition is most likely to take place in irreducible hernia or umbilical hernia, especially if the patient is constipated. As this condition develops the tumor enlarges and becomes tender and painful. The abdomen may become distended and painful. Soothing procedures are necessary until the bowels are emptied, by first giving an enema, and then, castor oil. Surgery is usually necessary to repair this type of hernia.

Inflamed hernia is due to injury of an irreducible hernia. It is a local peritonitis manifesting as a mass that is tender, painful and hot. In inflamed enterocele there is much fluid formed, while in epiplocele the mass becomes hard.

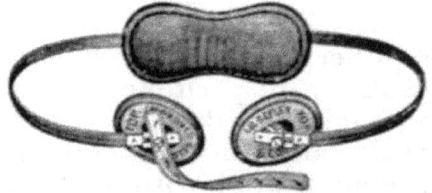

A Victorian double ball-and-socket type truss for a double hernia.

There is constipation, vomiting and usually fever. The hernia cannot be reduced, and the mass shows impulses on coughing. Every means possible should be employed to empty the bowels, using enema to first empty below the hernia, then giving castor oil or salts. Surgery is advisable to prevent strangulation.

Strangulated hernia is a condition in which the blood vessels, whether intestinal or omental, are constricted and blood circulation arrested along fecal obstruction. Strangulated hernia is dangerous to life. It usually occurs in patients having old inguinal hernia, who lead an active life. There may occur a slipping out of more intestine or omentum into the inguinal sac and this causes a pressure at the opening or neck of the sac, sufficient to check the blood circulation. The patient feels sharp colicky pains in the region of the umbilicus soon after this occurs and he rapidly grows weak. There is much retching and often, vomiting. The pain gradually becomes continuous. Later the hernia becomes irreducible. It is found larger than usual, tender, painful and the skin above it may be reddened. There is no impulse upon coughing.

This type of hernia usually results in gangrene with danger of death unless surgery is applied. Measures should be taken to reduce the condition. The patient is placed on his back, preferably on an incline plane with the body higher than the head, the knees bent to relax the abdomen as much as possible. By gentle manipulation it is frequently possible to reduce this condition. Then, the abdominal walls can be strengthened. If reduction is impossible, surgery is necessary.

Inguinal herniae are also named according to their contents. In *enterocele* the sac contains portions of intestine. In *epiplocele* the sac contains omentum. *Entero-epipocele* is the name applied when the sac contains both intestine and omentum. A *cystocele* contains a portion of the bladder.[45]

In his 1908 book *Hernia: Its Cause and Treatment*, Dr. Robert William Murray writes:

☛ When studying the etiology of abnormal or diseased conditions in man, it is often of great assistance to study similar or allied conditions as they occur in the lower animals. If inguinal hernia be considered from this point of view, new light may be thrown upon an old subject and some information obtained which may help us to answer the question we are now considering.

In the majority of mammals the testes pass out of the abdomen into the scrotum preceded by a fold of peritoneum, the processus vaginalis testis, which remains patent [open] throughout life. The anatomy of the muscular and aponeurotic structures forming the inguinal canal in scrotal mammalia is practically the same as in man.

There is apparently some relationship between the natural position of the animal's body, horizontal or vertical, and the patency or otherwise of the processus vaginalis testis. In quadrupeds this process invariably communicates with the general peritoneal cavity, and in rodents the channel of communication is so free as to allow the testes to pass periodically from the abdomen into the scrotum. In quadrumana, whose bodies are as frequently vertical as horizontal, the processus vaginalis is very narrow, offering a marked difference to what obtains in rodents, whilst in the higher apes the testes pass into the scrotum two or three days before birth and the processus vaginalis is normally completely obliterated.

I would particularly draw attention to the fact that in rodents the funicular process must be exceptionally wide to permit of the free passage of the testis, yet these animals do not suffer from inguinal hernia, pointing to the sphincter-like action of the muscles guarding the inguinal canal. Doubtless the high position of the inguinal canal in quadrupeds is the chief reason for the gut not entering it, and if rodents habitually adopted the practice of walking on their hind legs, a method of progression which was invariably adopted by the White Rabbit in *Alice in Wonderland*, oblique inguinal hernia would probably become of such frequent occurrence as to threaten the extinction of the species.

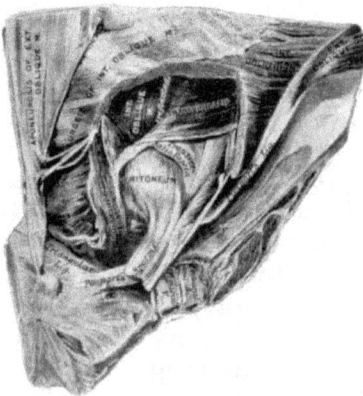

Dissection of an oblique inguinal hernia, showing its various coverings.

Hernia is by no means uncommonly seen in domesticated animals such as the horse, the cow, the dog, and the ass, but, of all domesticated animals, the horse is the one which has received the greatest amount of attention at the hands of veterinary surgeons, who are unanimously of opinion that the bowel in an ordinary inguinal hernia invariably descends into a sac which is of congenital origin. Inguinal hernia in the horse would probably be met with much more frequency than it is, on account of the patency of the funicular process, were it not that the inguinal canal occupies a position less exposed than is the case in man to the influence of gravity on the abdominal viscera. In this animal the great strength of the abdominal muscles and fascia which guard the inguinal opening also affords additional security in preventing the escape of the abdominal contents. Professor W. O. Williams, in his work on *Veterinary Surgery*, says:

> "Inguinal hernia is most frequently met with in stallions and young animals, and essentially consists in the passage of a fold of intestine into the inguinal canal through the internal abdominal ring. It is very frequently seen in India and on the Continent, but is uncommon in this country from the fact that stallions are not often used for working purposes. It is but rarely seen in the gelding, and scarcely ever in the mare, although it is possible that it may occur in both."

The importance of a patent funicular process in determining the occurrence of a hernia is well illustrated in the case of domesticated animals called upon to do work which in a sense is unnatural to them. In India and on the Continent stallions are used for working purposes, and they frequently suffer from inguinal hernia. On the other hand, inguinal hernia is rarely seen in the gelding, and yet it is the gelding that as a rule does the hardest work. Further, the operation for radical cure of inguinal hernia in the stallion consists essentially in excision of the sac after applying a ligature to the neck of it. No attempt is made to narrow the inguinal canal by suturing. This operation is attended by most satisfactory results, except when the animal is an old one or the hernia exceptionally large.

I think, then, *we may take it as an undoubted fact that in domesticated animals, such as the horse, the dog, and the cat, the sac of an inguinal hernia is of congenital origin and not acquired. The main factors in the causation of such a hernia are the presence of a patent funicular process, together with the want of power in the muscles guarding the internal abdominal ring* [my emphasis, L.S.]. In the case of a stallion used for draught purposes the muscles guarding the internal abdominal ring may be at times unduly strained, and thus the bowel is allowed to pass into the scrotum.

In the case of the dog I would suggest that the hernia appears because the muscles are deficient in tone, owing to the unnatural and indolent life many of these animals lead.[46]

Chapin Aaron Harris' 1855 *A Dictionary of Medical Terminology, Dental Surgery, and the Collateral Sciences*, defines hernia this way:

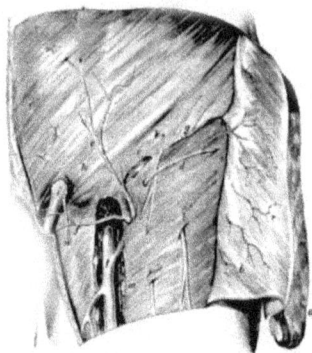

Superficial dissection of inguinal and crural regions. The front of the body is on the left.

☞ A tumor formed by the displacement and protrusion of the whole or part of a viscus. Hernia is distinguished according to the region in which it occurs. It is termed reducible, when it can be readily returned back into the abdomen; irreducible, when there is no constriction, yet from adhesion or its large size, it cannot be put back; and strangulated, or incarcerated, when its reduction is prevented by constriction. Hernia may exist from birth, or occur from accident or injury at any subsequent period of life. In the former case it is termed congenital, and in the latter accidental.[47]

Dr. Marcy defines a hernia like this:

☞ Hernia may be defined as the portion of the contents of any cavity projecting through an opening in its walls. However, surgically considered, unless otherwise stated, the term is usually restricted to the abdomen.

Abdominal herniæ are remarkable for their frequency, variety, and the danger attending them. They are produced by the protrusion of the viscera, contained in the abdomen, through the natural or accidental apertures, in the parietes of that cavity. The organs which form them most frequently are intestines and omentum.[48]

In his 1908 book *The Technic of Modern Operations for Hernia*, Dr. Alexander Hugh Ferguson writes:

☛ A hernia or rupture is the protrusion of any viscus from the cavity in which it is normally contained. The term is usually applied to protrusions of abdominal and pelvic viscera, although organs situated in other cavities may become herniated.

. . . The hernia may be a congenital or an acquired one. Its protrusion may occur through openings in the abdominal wall, which were present in fetal life and failed to close at birth, as, for instance, the umbilicus and the funicular process of the peritoneum. These are congenital hernias.

The protrusion also may occur at points where the abdominal wall is weaker than elsewhere, such as the inguinal region, where the spermatic cord passes through the inguinal canal; at the umbilicus, where the muscle tissue is naturally deficient; in the femoral region, where the large vessels and nerves pass out of the pelvis; and at other points where there is a normal diastasis of muscle fibers, the space being bridged over by connective tissue only, as in Petit's triangle, between the latissimus dorsi and the external oblique muscles, and in the diaphragm. Hernias occurring at these points are of the acquired variety.[49]

In his 1821 book entitled *A Treatise on the Radical Cure of Hernia or Rupture*, Dr. William Dufour described a hernia this way:

☛ Hernia is a disorderly protrusion of a part from the limit within which, in its original and natural state it was bounded or circumscribed. The English word is rupture, signifying that the part disordered is broken, or the effect of something broken forth from its natural limits. The parts subject to this disorderly protrusion, are generally the intestines, the fatty covering called the omentum, and the membrane called the peritoneum, which envelopes them.

. . . The internal belly, or peritoneum, is a mere bag, containing very flexible and easily moveable or shifting portions of the intestines, pressing upon its lowest parts, and upon each other; in a state of disease from relaxation or from debility, the muscles, membranes, or ligaments, which in a healthy state serve to retain this bag and its contents within their proper bounds, give way in one part, or they become imperfect; in either case a part of the bag with its contents protrudes. At certain parts or points, the muscles, membranes, or ligaments, are interrupted; orifices or openings for the better answering natural and economical purposes are left; through them, when their immediate boundaries are relaxed, a part of the bag with its proximate contents protrudes. The opening proper for the purposes above-mentioned, is technically called a ring, or the abdominal ring. Through this ring in men passes the vessels proper to the testicles. In order that nothing besides these vessels, with their accompaniments, may pass, the ring is covered, strengthened, and guarded by certain ligaments or parts of muscles, familiarly called straps. The outer skin, with these ligaments or straps, are called the parietes of the abdomen, that is to say, the walls or boundaries of the belly. In robust habits these are sufficient, but when from debility of constitution, from sedentary occupation, from over-exertion, or from any other cause, they shall, as observed above, have become relaxed or disordered, præternatural dilatation, or extension takes place, and through the ring before described, and stated to be designed to allow the passage of the vessels, a portion of intestine or gut, or of the omentum passes or protrudes. When the intestine or gut passes or protrudes, it has some analogy with the double finger of a glove, passing through a hole in a bag, already lined with linen or other material, and carrying before it such lining. When a portion of the omentum passes, it is by reason of its having been pushed through the orifice, or hole in the bag so lined, as stated above. And it very often happens that the omentum alone passes; yet, when the intestine passes a portion of the peritoneum, before described, must, as it is its natural covering, or envelope, common to the whole intestines, also pass.[50]

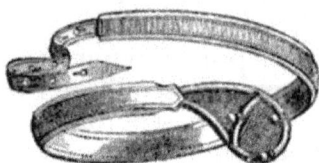

Victorian anatomical truss, anterior aspect.

In his 1906 book *General Surgery*, veterinarian Eugen Fröhner discusses the topics of the movability of the hernia's contents and herniological classification, both which are relevant to our study:

☛ **With reference to the mobility of the hernial contents, they are classified as reducible (moveable, free), that is, they may be pushed through the hernial mouth into the abdominal cavity; and irreducible (immoveable), that is, a hernia that cannot be returned. The immobility is due, either to adhesions between the hernial contents and the hernial sac, which is especially common in omental hernias (immobility of the omentum); to incarceration (constriction, strangulation) of the prolapsed viscera, this is especially frequent in intestinal hernias.**[51]

Dr. Fröhner goes on to define the all important symptoms of both a reducible hernia and an irreducible ("incarcerated") hernia from a veterinarian's viewpoint:

☛ **A reducible hernia is characterized by a large or small hernial swelling which occupies a characteristic seat in the umbilical or inguinal region, etc. The swelling is painless, is not characterized by a rise of temperature, and has a soft peculiar consistence; the skin is moveable on the surface, occasionally one may easily palpate intestinal loops or pieces of omentum at its base. Percussion occasion ally gives a tympanitic sound (air in the intestinal loops); on auscultation one can occasionally hear rumbling or gurgling peristaltic sounds. On pressure the swelling be comes smaller and finally entirely disappears in the abdominal cavity. Palpation of the abdominal wall reveals the hernial mouth, it varies in size from a pea to that of one's fist; in form it is round, oval or elongated; whenever a hernia has existed for a long time the free margin of ring becomes firm and tendinous. In rare cases the abdominal sac becomes ossified in cattle.**

Incarcerated hernia, especially in horses, is first recognized by colic (strangulated inguinal hernia of stallions); in dogs and swine one further observes vomiting, and even stercoraceous vomiting; constipation is present in all animals. On local examination one finds an inflammatory swelling at the seat of the hernial sac; attempts to return the hernial contents are unsuccessful.[52]

Human Anatomy

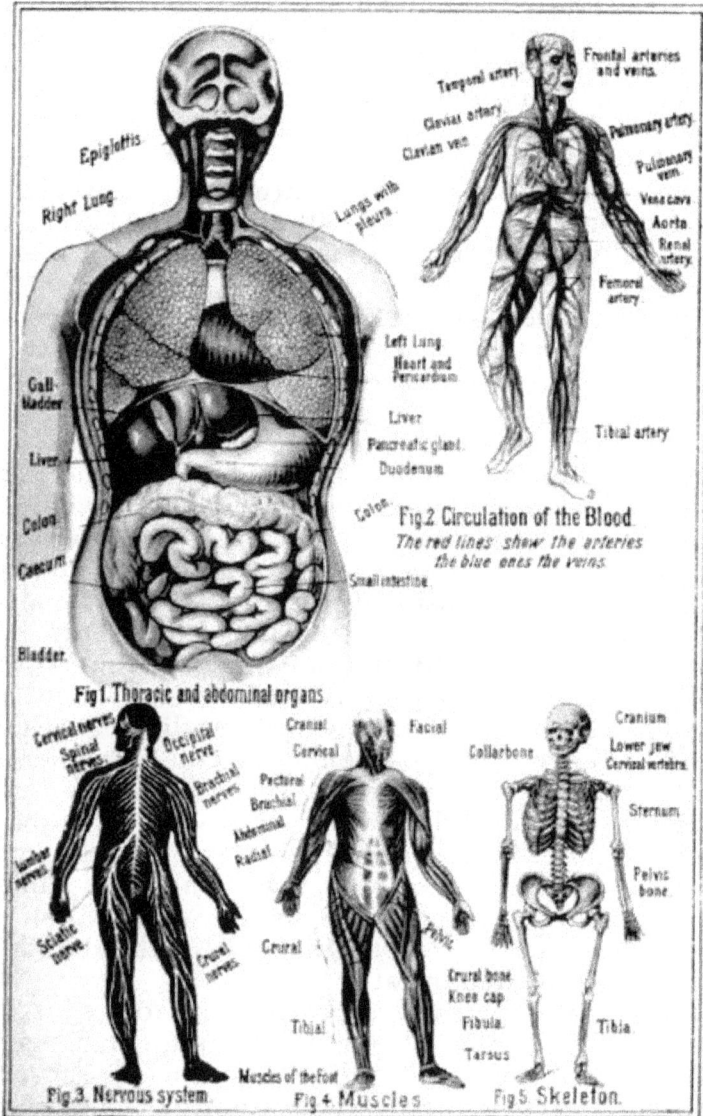

Showing the abdominal organs, blood circulation, nervous system, muscles, and skeleton.

DIAGNOSING REDUCIBLE INGUINAL HERNIA

Diagnosing a reducible inguinal hernia is fairly straightforward, as Charles E. Sajous writes in his 1904 book *Sajous's Analytical Cyclopedia of Practical Medicine*:

☛ **A reducible hernia usually presents the following signs: A soft tumor or swelling is found in one of the hernial openings; this swelling disappears on lying down, or on moderate pressure. It gives a distinct impulse on coughing, and usually it is seen to increase in size during the act of coughing or straining of the abdominal muscles.**[53]

Though externally determining which type of hernia one has, complete/direct or incomplete/oblique, can be difficult (if not often impossible):

☛ **There is one important clinical method which will nearly always enable one to make a positive diagnosis: After the hernia has been reduced, press two or three fingers over the internal ring, leaving the external ring free or uncovered. The patient is then asked to cough, and if the hernia is direct** [or complete], **it will emerge from the external ring; if it is oblique** [or incomplete], **the pressure over the internal ring will prevent its appearance. In some cases the diagnosis is very difficult, except by operation . . .**[54]

NOMENCLATURAL CHAOS & DISARRAY

In his 1908 essay, "Hernia," Dr. Coley (mentioned above) points out that there is no medical consensus on the definitions of the two primary hernial categories, congenital (genetically inherited) and acquired (sudden bodily trauma):

☛ **All hernias have been generally divided into two groups, i.e., congenital and acquired. These terms, however, have given rise to a great deal of confusion. Even now there is no well-settled rule as to their proper interpretation. Some writers class as congenital all hernial sacs which are preformed, calling acquired all sacs that have developed after birth. This would be an excellent rule, were it possible to apply it practically. Inasmuch as the only way of definitely telling that a sac** is preformed or of pre-natal origin is by the fact that it communicates with the tunica vaginalis testis, it has been a rule with most writers to class as congenital hernias only such as showed this connection. This test, however, rules out not only a very large number of sacs in the male, in which by reason of the appearance of a hernia in earliest infancy the presence of a preformed sac is practically proved, but it also rules out all cases of inguinal hernia in the female. To thus restrict the term "congenital" to a comparatively small proportion of cases, in the male is, I believe, most misleading. It is probable that in the vast majority of inguinal hernias in the male, and practically all in the female, the sac is preformed, i.e., there is an open funicular process of peritoneum

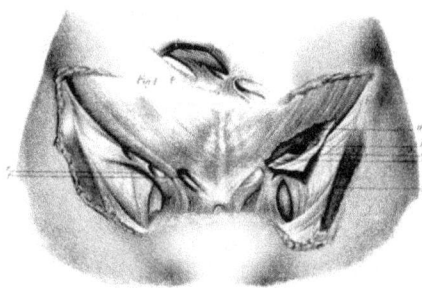

Surgical anatomy of inguinal hernia, showing pertinent muscles, cords, rings, arches, and natural openings.

existing at birth, even though the hernia may not develop until adult life. The principal exception to this broad generalization would be the direct hernias. This variety of hernia more accurate knowledge has shown to be far less frequent than has hitherto been supposed. My own operative statistics show 39 cases of direct hernia in a total of over 1950 operations. Of these, only two occurred in the female.[55]

The importance of Dr. Coley's statements concerning the focus of this book—namely, non-surgical self-treatment of inguinal hernia—will become more apparent in the next chapter.

ADDITIONAL IMPORTANT HERNIAL DATA
Let us add to our hernial knowledge with the following comments from a 1920 article, "Some Pertinent Thoughts Relating to Hernia," by Dr. A. Wiese Hammer:

☛ Inguinal hernias are divided into the Direct, which are always *acquired*, and the Indirect or Oblique, which may be *congenital* or *acquired*. Indirect inguinal hernia [also known as "external hernia"] constitutes 97 percent of all inguinal hernias, and here at the outset, an effort will be made to clarify the terms, congenital and infantile, which are so frequently confused. The hernia may descend into the unobliterated processus vaginalis, either in the male or female, being then called *congenital* hernia, or into a sac formed by the protruded peritoneum of the abdomen—*acquired* hernia.[56]

In his 1889 book *A Treatise on Hernia: The Radical Cure by the Use of the Buried Antiseptic Animal Suture*, Dr. Henry Orlando Marcy gives a wonderful description of the abdominal environment in which inguinal hernias develop:

☛ The construction of the abdominal walls is a beautiful example of nature's marvelous adaptability of means to the end to be subserved. The abdomen must be always full, no matter how varied its contents, and subject to equable pressure. The amount of pressure varies with contents, position of the body, and muscular contractility of the abdominal walls. For obvious reason, the tension is greatest at the lowest portion of any supporting cavity. This would be the pelvic basin but for the disposition of the bony structure of the trunk, where the relation of the incline of the brim of the pelvis to the projection of the sacrum throws the abdominal weight forward, and lessens materially the strain upon the floor of the pelvis.[57]

In his 1878 book *The Principles and Practice of Surgery*, Dr. Hayes Agnew recorded this description of hernias:

☛ [A hernia] . . . is the protrusion of an intestine, of omentum [a fold of the peritoneum], or of both, from the interior to the exterior of the abdominal cavity, in the course of certain blood-vessels. The abdominal walls, for the most part, are admirably constructed to prevent visceral protrusions. They consist of stratifications of muscular and aponeurotic tissues, the fibres of which are disposed in different directions. The external oblique muscles run from above downwards; the internal oblique, from below upwards; the transversalis, transversely; and the recti, with their tendinous intersections and sheaths of strong fibrous tissue, extend perpendicularly between the pelvis and thorax. There are, however, certain points in the parietes [walls] which are necessarily less capable of resisting pressure from within than others; and these points correspond to where the blood vessels designed to supply the outstanding organs leave the body. A knowledge of these vessels is the key to a proper understanding of hernia.

General Division of Hernia.—There are two grand divisions of hernia, congenital and acquired. Under the first division are included all herniae that occur before birth; under the second, all that result from weakness of the abdominal parietes or from accident after birth.

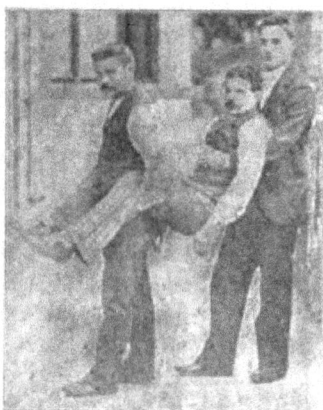

Man with an inguinal hernia being transported to a medical facility.

Varieties of Hernia.—When a hernia follows the course of the spermatic cord or blood-vessels, it is called a spermatic or an inguinal hernia; when it takes the direction of the femoral or crural vessels, it constitutes a femoral or a crural hernia; when its direction is in the course of the umbilical vessels, it is termed an umbilical hernia; if in the course of the obturator arteries, it is an obturator hernia; if it follows the gluteal or ischiatic vessels, it constitutes a gluteal or ischiatic hernia. The last three forms are very rare. In addition to these varieties, there are a number of herniæ which do not follow, in all cases, the course of the blood-vessels. They are the diaphragmatic, the pudendal, the perineal, and the sacro-rectal herniæ.[58]

VARIETIES & TYPES OF HERNIA

How many types of hernias are recognized by the medical establishment? It depends on what time period one is looking at. In 1921, for example, under the direction of Surgeon General Hugh Smith Cumming, the U.S. government compiled the following official list of 31 varieties:

Hernia, diaphragmatic.
Hernia, diverticulum of intestine.
Hernia, epigastric.
Hernia, epigastric, strangulated.
Hernia, femoral.
Hernia, femoral, strangulated.
Hernia, inguinal, external or oblique.
Hernia, inguinal, external or oblique, strangulated.
Hernia, inguinal, funicular.
Hernia, inguinal, internal or direct.
Hernia, inguinal, internal or direct, strangulated.
Hernia, into lesser peritoneal sac.

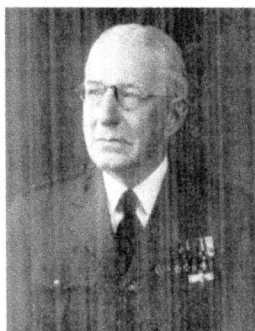

Hernia, ischiatic.
Hernia, ischiatic, strangulated.
Hernia, ischiorectal.
Hernia, ischiorectal, strangulated.
Hernia, lumbar.
Hernia, lumbar, strangulated.
Hernia, obturator.
Hernia, obturator, strangulated.
Hernia, of muscle.
Hernia, perineal.
Hernia, retroperitoneal.
Hernia, sciatic.
Hernia, umbilical.
Hernia, umbilical, strangulated.
Hernia, ventral.

Hugh S. Cumming.

Hernia, ventral, postoperative.
Hernia, ventral, strangulated.
Hernia (otherwise unclassified).
Hernia, strangulated (otherwise unclassified).[59]

DISTINGUISHING A HERNIA FROM A RUPTURE

In his 1864 work *Medical Common Sense; Applied to the Causes, Prevention and Cure of Chronic Diseases and Unhappiness in Marriage*, Dr. Edward B. Foote writes:

☞ It is a common error to suppose that rupture and hernia are two names for one disease. Rupture, properly speaking, is when the intestines or other organs unnaturally protrude or intrude through *lacerated or broken walls or membranes*, which, in health, retain them. Hernia is an abnormal protrusion or intrusion of the intestines or other organs through *natural apertures or canals* which have become relaxed or enlarged [my emphasis, L.S.]. They may be called protrusions when they exhibit themselves externally, and intrusions when they invade one or more of the internal cavities. (I make this distinction with the full knowledge that the term hernia is derived from a Greek word signifying *protrusion from*.) If the protruding or intruding parts can be replaced, then it is called reducible rupture or hernia; if they cannot be restored to their natural position, they bear the name of irreducible rupture or hernia. The latter is usually a painful and dangerous disease, and the former may suddenly become so, for if, at any time, a sudden protrusion should be accompanied with a constriction of the aperture or canal through which it passes, what is called strangulated rupture or hernia ensues, and unless immediate relief is obtained, a hectic flush, vomiting, obstinate constipation, rapid pulse, etc., usher in the fatal stage of the disease, which is characterized by a distended and hard condition of the abdomen, cold extremities, clammy sweats, hiccough, sinking pulse, etc.

Rupture more commonly takes place somewhere about the abdomen, and may be caused by a violent blow, a fall, heavy lifting or pregnancy. Unless the skin is broken (which seldom happens) as well as the inner walls of the abdomen, the protrusion presents very much the appearance of a common tumor. But, if reducible, it may be removed by gentle pressure or by reclining on the back, while coughing, sneezing, reaching upward; and even standing erect gives it unusual prominence.

Hernia most commonly makes its appearance in males, in what is called the inguinal region. [This region is located in the groin and is transversed by the inguinal canal.] A similar canal exists in the opposite groin. It must be understood that beneath the skin, the intestines are confined in their proper position by three layers of membrane, muscle, etc., which are denominated the walls of the abdomen. Through slits, commonly called rings, in these, pass the inguinal canals from the rings in the inner walls to the scrotum. . . . The distance from the internal to the external ring, is usually about two inches; through these rings and canals on either side, the testicles descend to the scrotum, in most cases, just before, or soon after birth, although the descension does not, in some cases, take place till a much later period. After the descension of the testicles, these canals become the residence of the spermatic cords, and not unfrequently, the location of hernial tumors. . . .

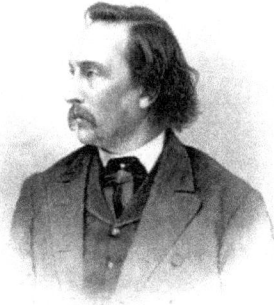

Dr. Edward B. Foote.

Females sometimes have inguinal hernia. Those canals which constitute the paths of the descending testicles and spermatic cords in the male, are occupied, in the female, by small ligaments to steady the womb and prevent its turning backward. But they are so much smaller in females, this description of hernia seldom afflicts women. Occasionally a case of this kind is met with, and now and then, one in which the protrusion descends to the labiæ [labium].[60]

Due to the confusion caused by, as well as the inappropriate use of, the word rupture, Dr. William Burton De Garmo wrote the following in his 1907 book *Abdominal Hernia: Its Diagnosis and Treatment*:

☞ The word "rupture," so commonly used to denote a condition of hernia, will be, as far as possible, avoided in this work, as it leads to an erroneous impression of what actually occurs. In the early ages this term was applied under the supposition that there was actual rupture [tearing] of the peritoneum. It is now well known that there is rarely laceration of tissue hernia results, in almost every instance, from the gradual stretching of tissue and escape of the abdominal contents, either into a preformed (congenital) sac, or by the formation of a sac (acquired) from the peritoneal lining of the abdomen.[61]

In his 1900 book *Hernia: Its Etiology, Symptoms and Treatment*, Dr. William McAdam Eccles writes:

☞ The word "rupture," although no doubt used to denote protrusions through the abdominal wall, is open to the very serious objection that it implies—at any rate, in the lay mind—an altogether mistaken idea of the cause of the swelling. In the majority of cases a hernia is of gradual and slow formation, and this without any tearing or breaking of tissue, such as is clearly indicated in the use of the word "rupture."[62]

Likewise, in 1920 Dr. Hammer writes:

☛ This seems an appropriate place to condemn the term "rupture" as a synonym of hernia. This lay expression was early employed to meet the fallacious notion that a hernia resulted from a tearing or bruising of the musculature or was a direct result of violence, leading to an extrusion of the intestines. Instead of these crude explanations, *today we know that the chief cause of hernia is some congenital defect, which assumes a more concrete form through some one or other exciting causes* [my emphasis, L.S.].[63]

Victorian scientists observed this same phenomenon in livestock, particularly horses, as veterinarian Dr. John A. W. Dollar notes in his 1912 book *Regional Veterinary Surgery and Operative Technique*:

☛ In stallions with abnormally wide abdominal rings, and less frequently in geldings, the small intestine or omentum may enter the inguinal canal. . . . *Inguinal hernia is generally congenital . . . The tendency to it seems to be inherited* [my emphasis, L.S.]. Its production is favoured by all circumstances which cause increased abdominal pressure, such as tympanites, severe exertion, hard drawing on soft ground (where the action of the muscles in lifting the feet also produces dilatation of the abdominal ring), or struggling in hobbles.[64]

In his 1921 book *The Principles and Practice of Surgery*, Herman A. Haubold writes:

☛ A hernia may be defined as a protrusion of one or more of the abdominal viscera through a normal or an abnormal opening. *The chief* [i.e., main] *cause of hernia of this sort is a congenital defect, while the exciting cause plays a minor part* [my emphasis, L.S.].[65]

In 1884, in *The International Encyclopedia of Surgery*, Dr. John Wood offers these thoughts:

☛ **Most frequently the opening** [out of which an inguinal hernia protrudes] **is constituted by the enlargement of a natural aperture between the muscles and fascia. Such protrusions are named according to their situation:** *Hernia inguinalis, Hernia cruralis vel femoralis, Hernia umbilicalis, Hernia obturatoria, Hernia sacro-sciatica.* **All these pass through dilatations of natural openings, and are covered by the integuments and abdominal fascia varying with their position.**[66]

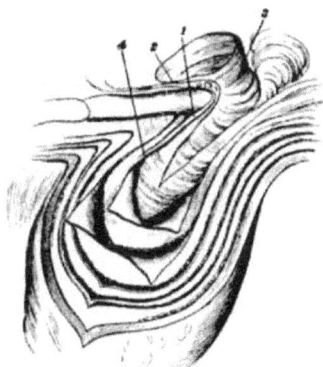

Diagram of inguinal hernia, showing various coverings.

INGUINAL HERNIAS TEND TO OCCUR AT "WEAK POINTS"

The idea that many if not most inguinal hernias are the result of a natural aperture or opening in genetically "weak areas" in the abdomen rather than from tearing of the abdominal tissue was not original to the Victorian Age. In 1701 a man named Dr. Mery published his observation that in the formation of a hernia, **"the peritoneum was not torn, but simply stretched."**[67] Around 1730, French physician Michel-Louis Reneaulme de Lagaranne and French surgeon Rene Jacques Croissant de Garengeot proposed that:

☛ **. . . the intestines were subjected to pressure upon all sides by the abdominal muscles and diaphragm, from which they attempted to escape through the weak portions of the abdominal wall, particularly in those places which give exit to the vessels.**[68]

Likewise, in 1916 Dr. Bevan writes of the **"common forms of hernia,"** which are

☛ **due to congenital defects at three** *weak points* [my emphasis, L.S.] **in the abdominal wall—the inguinal region, the femoral region, and the umbilical region.**[69]

In his 1870 book *A System of Practical Surgery*, Sir William Fergusson writes:

☞ *The anatomist is familiar with all the weak points in the* *parietes* [walls] *of the abdomen through which protrusions,* *constituting herniæ, make their appearance* [my emphasis, L.S.]. **At the groins, in the inguinal and crural canals, at various parts in the pelvis, at the umbilicus, and at other parts, or where wounds, if neglected, are likely to be followed by protrusion, he can have no difficulty in appreciating the leading features in such cases. By far the most common are those at the inguinal and crural canals, and at the umbilicus . . .**[70]

ABDOMINAL WEAKNESS NOT EXTERNAL INJURY
Clearly, the main cause of nearly all inguinal hernias is an inherited weakness in the abdominal wall, not trauma.[71] Trauma can sometimes be the *immediate* or *exciting* cause, but it is much less likely to be the *precipitating* or *main* cause, as T. Henry Walnut writes in his 1925 article, "Hernia as a Compensable Accident Under the Workman's Compensation Act of Pennsylvania":

☞ **Returning to the discussion of inguinal hernias, which constitute, as already pointed out, by far, the largest number that occur, we should understand that direct inguinal hernias are, of course, not caused by open funicular canals; according to Coley, they are due to a weakness of structures which surround the external ring, while Blake would ascribe them to a weakness in the transversalis fascia in a triangular space, bounded above by the fibres of the internal oblique, internally by the rectus and below by Pouparts ligament. He calls it the "undefended space".**
      . . . The reason for this prevalence of indirect inguinal hernia is a weakness in the abdominal wall at a point known as the internal ring of the inguinal canal. Pressure of the abdominal contents upon this point forces a portion of the contents into the canal.
      . . . Berger states that we know that hernia is, in the great majority of cases, not the result of an accident. Though accidental or professional effort may occasionally be the cause, a hernia is usually the result of a slow process, the true origin of which is a constitutional

[i.e., an inherent part of the body] defect of the abdominal walls. It may be a congenital feebleness, consisting of malformation or weakness of the hernial orifices, the appearance of the hernia depending upon the gradual weakening of the aponeurosis or muscular plane. Under the

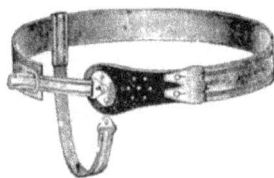

Victorian elastic truss with hard rubber front plate.

influence of normal effort increasingly repeated, these weak places become enlarged and the hernia is produced. In some cases the accident reveals a condition which may have been long present, but was hitherto unsuspected. The accident, then, is not the first, and perhaps not the principal cause, but may have hastened the development of a condition which, otherwise, would not have occurred for some time, perhaps never.[72]

Likewise, Victorian and early 20th-Century veterinarians found that inguinal hernias in their animal patients were usually the result of organs poking through a natural opening in the abdomen (actually bands of muscles),[73] not a "tear" in the tissues. Writing in 1926 in *A Study of Hernia in Swine*, Dr. Bruce Lester Warwick notes:

☛ Inguinal hernia is that form of hernia in which one or more loops of the intestines or other abdominal organs pass through the abdominal wall at or alongside of the inguinal canal. This canal is the passageway through which the spermatic cord normally extends in the boar.
  There is a slit-like opening in the abdominal wall, situated between the edge of one of the abdominal muscles (the internal oblique) and a ligament (the inguinal) which lies behind the canal. The inguinal canals are situated one on each side of the penis about midway between the scrotum and the free end of the sheath.[74]

DESCRIBING THE PARTS OF A HERNIA
What are the parts constituting a hernia? Dr. Eccles responds with the following:

☛ A fully-formed hernia consists of (1) a sac; and (2) its contents.

1. Sac:
   (a) Mouth.
   (b) Neck.
   (c) Body.
2. Contents:
   (a) Omentum.
   (b) Intestine.
   (c) Other Viscera.
   (d) Fluid.

1. The Sac of a Hernia—This is formed by a protrusion of parietal peritoneum. It is made up of three parts, viz., the mouth of the sac, the neck, and the body.

The mouth of the sac is the aperture by which its interior communicates with the peritoneal cavity. In the early stages of the formation of the sac the mouth is the widest part, but as the process of peritoneum is further and further protruded, so the mouth becomes smaller and narrower in comparison with the rest of the sac. The neck of the sac is the constricted portion which is between the mouth and the body. It is for the most part found lying in tissues of the abdominal wall. In the beginning of the formation of the sac the portion constituting its neck will be probably thrown into folds.

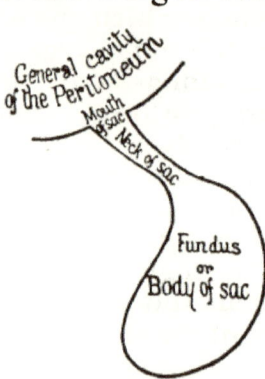

The parts of a hernial sac.

The body of the sac is that expanded portion which protrudes beyond the aperture in the abdominal wall. The body, which is often termed the fundus, may be pyriform or globular in shape, and it varies very much in size. The sac is said to have vessels ramifying over it in an arborescent manner; but it must be confessed that these vessels are often but very poorly marked.

The formation of the sac of an acquired hernia is somewhat difficult to satisfactorily account for. In the very early periods of its development, on account of the intra-abdominal pressure being suddenly increased, a slight bulging may occur in the region of a weak spot in the abdominal wall. This is more easily seen than palpated. On the pressure being removed, the parietal peritoneum returns to its normal relations. If, however, the same conditions be many times repeated, there comes a period when the membrane will have yielded so much as to remain permanently bulged. The process of peritoneum thus formed may be caused partly by displacement of peritoneum, or partly by the gradual stretching of the portion of the membrane involved. At first there is but little adhesion of the sac to the tissues into which it is protruded, and it may be occasionally possible to dislocate it from its surroundings and return it within the abdominal wall. Very rapidly, however, the sac-wall tends to become firmly fixed in its new bed, and tedious dissection will be necessary to separate it from the structures outside it.

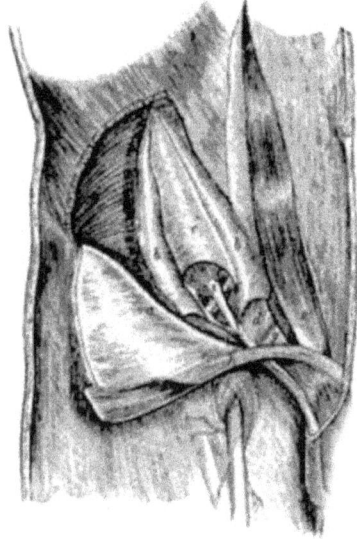

Deep dissection of inguinal canal and abdominal wall, showing many of the muscles, ligaments, fascia, tendons, fibers, openings, and rings associated with inguinal hernia.

Thus it will be seen that the formation of the sac of a hernia is a slow process, for the parietal peritoneum will neither stretch nor prolapse sufficiently to produce a sac in a day, or even a week or two; in fact, it usually takes months for the sac to be really apparent. It therefore follows, seeing that a hernial sac is not formed suddenly, that a fully developed acquired hernia, consisting as it does of a sac and its contents, cannot be created in a few hours.[75]

With this understanding of the Victorian view of hernial anatomy, we are now ready to survey the 19th-Century explanations for the causes behind hernias.

Healthy Food Plants

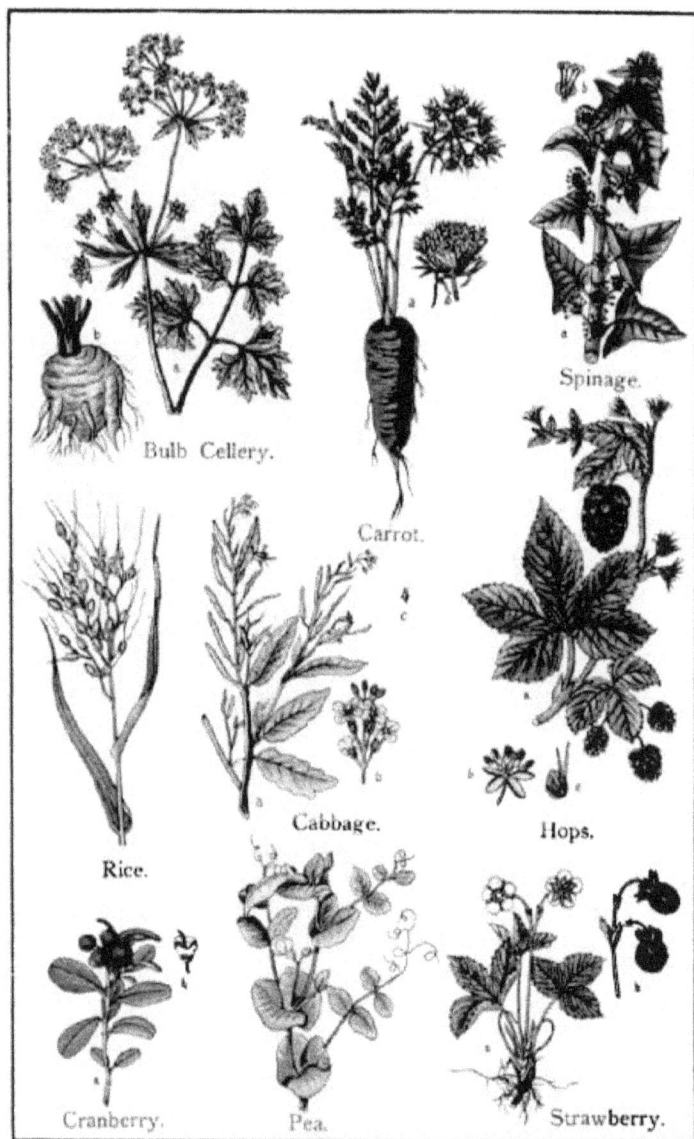

Edible vegetation used by Victorians to improve fitness and help heal inguinal hernia.

2

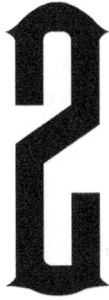

VICTORIAN EXPLANATIONS OF CAUSES OF INGUINAL HERNIA

HERNIOLOGICAL CAUSALITY

Confusion not only surrounds the definition of a hernia, but also what causes it, as was hinted at in the previous chapter. In 1900 Dr. Eccles opined:

☛ As to the causes of hernia, it must be confessed that even yet but little is known on this subject which may be considered as definite.[76]

Whatever the actual cause, an inguinal hernia, or "rupture," as some Victorian doctors mistakenly called it, can "happen" to anyone, at anytime, at any age, for almost any reason, or for no discernable reason. In 1821, in his book *A Treatise on the Radical Cure of Hernia or Rupture*, Dr. William Dufour writes:

☛ Rupture is a disease that from neither sex withholds its visitation. Neither is any period of life exempt from its coming on. Those who may otherwise boast of their strength, and those who may be otherwise than strong are subject to rupture; the robust and the puny, the labourer and him who has not laboured; the active; the quiescent; the rich; the poor; the noble; the gentle.[77]

COMMON CAUSES
In 1907 Dr. De Garmo listed a few of the more common causes:

(1) Constipation; (2) Vomiting; (3) Cough; (4) Lifting; (5) Shouting; (6) Posture; (7) Obstructions to urination; (8) Crying in children; (9) Acites [an effusion of fluid that collects in spaces within the abdomen].[78]

To this list Dr. Eccles adds: occupation, pregnancy, diseases of the lungs, straining during urination (known as micturition), straining at toilet, tight-lacing, and increase of bulk of the viscera.[79] As already mentioned, an enlarged prostate can also cause a hernia.[80]

CAUSE OFTEN UNKNOWN
On the other hand, unless you suffer an extreme and obvious bodily trauma—such as a severe blow to the abdomen—it is most likely that you will never know the cause of your hernia. Indeed, in many cases, sometimes well over 50 percent, the cause of a hernia cannot be determined by either the patient or their doctor. In 1908 Dr. Coley reported that:

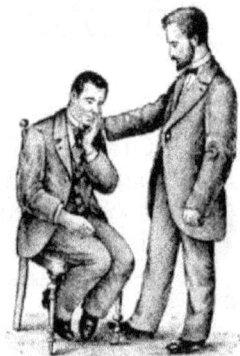

☛ **[In a recent hospital analysis,] . . . of 502 cases of umbilical hernia in female adults, in 204 no known cause could be assigned to the development of the rupture. . . . Of 4780 cases of hernia in adult males, over fifteen years of age, . . . 3102 [patients] stated that the rupture appeared without any known cause.**[81]

An inguinal hernia can negatively impact an individual's life in many ways.

PREDISPOSITION TO HERNIA
In his 1876 book *A Treatise on Hernia*, Greensville Dowell writes:

☛ **Many conditions predispose to hernia, such as sex, age, inheritance and conditions in life, which more or less predispose the patient to the inciting causes, as relaxation of the muscles, relaxation of the rings, general debility and obesity. The local predisposing causes are wounds, weakening the walls, burns, abscesses, ovarian tumors, ascites, punctures of surgical instruments, as** paracentesis abdominis, gastrotomy; the removal of tumors from the external wall.[82]

The reasons for tissue poking through the abdominal wall are indeed varied, numerous, and complex. In 1908 Dr. Murray writes:

☛ The ancients considered that hernia was due to a rupture of certain structures forming the abdominal wall, and the term "rupture" as applied to hernia still survives. Later writers realised that the peritoneum was stretched and not ruptured, and that the opening in the abdominal wall was caused by a separation or stretching of these structures, not by a tearing of the part.
. . . Though inguinal hernia is a very common complaint, has a wide geographical distribution and a very ancient origin [according to Medieval physician Prospero Alpini, it was "prevalent" 5,000 years ago in ancient Egypt][83]—in fact, it is far from improbable that an inguinal hernia first appeared in one of the children or grandchildren of Adam—we are still far from agreed as to its exact causation, and, consequently, still further from agreement as to the best way of curing it.[84]

Why do some individuals acquire a hernia while others do not? Dr. Murray answers the question this way:

☛ . . . I would suggest that the occurrence or not of a hernia largely depends upon two factors—the size of the opening at the internal abdominal ring and the strength of the muscles guarding it.
It is unnecessary for me to enter into anatomical details as to the formation of the inguinal canal and the attachment of the internal oblique and transversalis muscles, which together with Poupart's ligament form a sphincter-like structure guarding the canal. When the processus vaginalis is patent,[85] provided the opening at the internal abdominal ring is small and the muscles guarding it powerful, then the probability of a hernia occurring is slight. If, on the other hand, the internal opening is large and the inguinal sphincter weak, the probability of a hernia occurring is considerable.
. . . The frequency with which inguinal hernia first

appears about the age of puberty I would account for by the increased amount of exercise usually indulged in at this period, and the muscles which under ordinary conditions are able to guard the internal opening are suddenly over-taxed, and the bowel enters the inguinal canal. The escape of the bowel will, of course, largely depend upon the size of the internal opening.

When a hernia appears later in life, it may be even in old age, the same reasoning would hold good. Though the processus vaginalis testis has been to some extent patent since birth, no hernia has appeared because the opening at the internal abdominal ring was never large, and the inguinal muscles well able to guard it, but with declining years the weakened muscles gradually yield, and the bowel or omentum passes through.[86]

RELAXATION OF THE ABDOMINAL WALL & MUSCLES
In his 1898 book *The Natural Method of Healing*, Dr. Friedrich Eduard Bilz writes about the causes of hernias. Note that he appears to use the word "rupture" to mean the "widening of an opening" rather than by its true meaning, an actual "tear" in the tissue:

☛ The original cause of abdominal hernia is the relaxation of the abdominal wall and muscles, tissues etc., which in consequence are not only liable to fatty degeneration and distention, whereby an inherited or contracted tendency to rupture may be promoted and especially in those parts between the os pubis and the upper thigh where nature has left two fissures or openings, which are formed of elastic, tendonous muscular tissue, ligaments and sinews which are collectively known under the name of Aporiurosis, the inguinal canal which is embedded between the tissues of the broad, i.e., the internal slanting cross muscle of the abdomen, and also takes its course, for a short distance between these, at the same time serving as a passage-way for the spermatic cords in the male and the round ligaments in the female. Furthermore must be mentioned the crural canal through which the femoral arteries pass. All these parts may

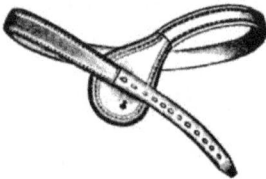
Victorian French truss.

become the seat of hernia, when a relaxed state exists in the respective internal (aponeurosis) and external (muscles) tissues etc., in consequence of one's landing on the heels after a leap, a fall upon the seat [buttocks], a violent fit of coughing or sneezing, a tight belt, tight-lacing, etc., whereby the entrails are pressed downwards, and easily produces a rupture.[87]

An early and very interesting description of the causes of inguinal hernias comes from Dr. Arnaud in 1748:

☛ Observations convince us, that these hernias are form'd by the dilatation of the peritoneum alone, and never by ruptures, unless they are produced by blows.
. . . The particular causes of these hernias in men, as well as in women, arise from this, that the ringlets are situated in the lowest part of the abdomen. In this low position they continually receive the matter of the internal perspiration, which is by little and little accumulated upon the division which separates the abdomen from the pelvis. The transpired matter, which, like an insensible vapour, is incessantly discharged from the parts contain'd in the abdomen, is indeed again received by the resorbent pores; but it is also sometimes discharged in a greater quantity, than that it can be received by these parts. In this case it must necessarily be accumulated, and remain in the lowest part of the abdomen. The peritoneum forms in this place, opposite to the ringlets, angular foldings, like small boats, proper for retaining and preserving this amass'd humidity. In consequence of this, the peritoneum and ringlets of the abdominal muscles must necessarily be relax'd, extend themselves, and yield to the efforts which the intestines make to descend, when the determining causes begin to act. A great many other causes, peculiar to hernias of the groin, contribute to their formation; but it is sufficient to have explain'd this, which is the principal, in order to discover the others, a detail of which would be too tedious. 'Tis, however, necessary to explain how the difference happens between the complete and incomplete hernia.
If the ringlet does not yield with too much ease, and if the peritoneum is but moderately elongated, the hernia

is incomplete; that is to say, it only forms a small eminence in form of an hemisphere, whose base is towards the abdomen, and its surface round. It remains in the flexure of the groin for a certain time, till by some new effort the parts are determined to descend farther. Then it becomes a complete hernia, because the parts finding no resistance, it has the liberty of descending into the scrotum, or the labia pudendi. It changes its figure, and, from round, becomes more and more long, in proportion to the progress of its descent.[88]

VIOLENT EXERTIONS

In 1864 Dr. Foote describes the causes of hernias in adults this manner:

☞ In adults, hernia is caused by violent exertions, lifting, straining at stool, severe coughing, convulsive sneezing, [etc.]. . . . Debility, arising from nervous derangements or blood impurities, either or both, may be safely pronounced the predisposing cause. The muscular system relaxed by debility, completely prepares the natural apertures through which pass the naval cord, the blood vessels of the thighs and the inguinal canals, for letting through the intestines or the omentum, or both. Whenever any tumors appear about the

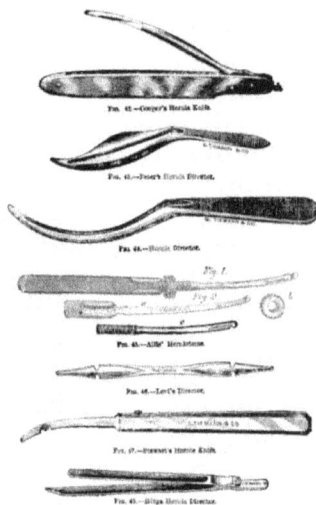

A hernia surgeon's tools of the trade.

abdomen, groins or thighs, notice should at once be taken whether they recede by manipulation or lying down, and if they do, there can be scarcely a doubt that they are tumors of a hernial nature. The individual so affected, male or female, should then lose no time in adopting means for their cure, for unless they are at least protected by a good truss, they may at any moment assume a dangerous form and imperil the life of the sufferer.[89]

FIRST & SECONDARY CAUSES
In 1878 Dr. Agnew depicts the causes of hernias in the following
description:

☛ **The causes of hernia are** *predisposing* **and** *exciting*.
1) *Predisposing.*—Among the predisposing causes may
be enumerated the following:
Muscular weakness of the abdominal parietes.—This is
often associated with a large accumulation of fat. This
weakness may be produced by wounds; by the atrophy
which follows protracted illness; by distention from large
accumulations of ascitic fluid, and from pregnancy; and
by a variety of other causes, such as coughing, straining,
jumping, vomiting, and lifting heavy weights.
Occupation.—The laboring classes, being the most
numerous, furnish the largest number of herniæ.
Occupations which require much physical effort when
the body is in the stooping posture expose most to the
disease, as the walls of the abdomen being thus relaxed
are less able to resist the pressure of the viscera. The
common habit among laborers of girding the loins tends
to produce the disease. It has been said that musicians
who use wind-instruments are much exposed to rupture.
This does not correspond with my observation. Persons
following this calling execute their music in the erect
position, and during the act of blowing the diaphragm is
gradually ascending, allowing the viscera of the abdomen
to rise. Gymnasts and contortionists might be supposed
to be particularly liable to hernia, yet this class of persons
are remarkably free from the disease. Indeed, the more I
observe of hernia the less importance do I attach to
occupation in the production of the malady.
Sex.—Males suffer more than females,—the
proportion, it is said, being four of the former to one of
the latter. This statement is based upon a report of the
London Truss Society, in which it appears that out of
96,886 persons applying for trusses only 18,492 were
females.
2) *Exciting cause.*—The exciting cause of hernia is
muscular action, by which, in certain postures of the
body, the viscera are forcibly thrust against the lower
portion of the abdomen, which yields at those points
naturally weakened by the passage of blood-vessels.

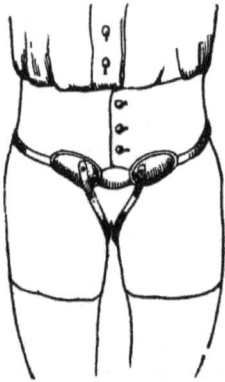

A Victorian illustration of Hirsch's Truss, with elastic bands.

Manner of occurrence.— Sometimes when a person is making an extraordinary muscular effort, or when an accident occurs in which an individual is thrown forcibly from a vehicle, the protrusion may be the work of an instant; but these are exceptional cases, the usual process being a gradual and slow one, requiring several months before the swelling has attained sufficient bulk or importance to attract attention particularly.

Symptoms of hernia.—There are certain signs common to all varieties of hernia, which may be enumerated as follows:

1. The presence of a swelling in certain defined localities, known as hernial regions; as in the region of the cord, the scrotum, the groin, or the umbilicus.

2. The swelling is usually painless, without unusual heat, and presents no discoloration.

3. The swelling is not fixed or permanent, but recedes and disappears entirely in the recumbent position,—or, at least, can be readily pressed back into the abdomen,—and reappears when the erect position is assumed.

4. In the act of coughing, a distinct impulse can be felt by the hand when placed over the tumor, and in the effort of straining or crying, a sudden enlargement will be observed in its size.

5. When the contents of the sac are entirely intestinal, the tumor will be elastic to the feel, resonant on percussion, and when returned will recede quickly in its entirety, and with a distinct gurgling sound or "flop." When the contents of the sac are exclusively omental, there will be an absence of resonance and of elasticity; there will be no sensible impulse communicated to the swelling either on straining or coughing; the tumor will have a doughy feel, and can only be restored, a small portion at a time, by taxis [manual manipulation]. When the intestines are distended by gaseous accumulations, no alteration of form occurs in the tumor. Omental hernia is

most common on the left side.

6. When both intestine and omentum occupy the sac, the characteristic signs of each will be present, but so blended and modified that it will be difficult to determine with certainty by the touch the existence of both.[90]

DISSECTING THE INGUINAL HERNIA
In his 1916 Dr. Gour makes these educational comments on the definition, description, and causes of hernias:

☛ There are many forms of hernia, but the inguinal type is the most common and most amenable to treatment. The term "rupture," so commonly used, is wrong. Rupture means an actual tearing of the peritoneum. In hernia there is seldom a tear, but we find a stretching of the natural openings of the inguinal canal through which the intestines or other tissues protrude. It is interesting to know how the term rupture originated.

R. W. Murray . . . says that "Galen (A.D. 131-201), whose knowledge of the body was based upon monkey anatomy, stated that inguinal hernia was due to a rupture of the peritoneal process, or to a gradual distention of it. In the case of rupture, it was believed that the tear involved the aponeurosis of the abdominal muscles as well as of the peritoneum. It is a strong evidence of the master mind of Galen that his anatomical and physiological teaching should have remained unchallenged until Vesalius (1514-1561), after carefully dissecting many human bodies, exposed the numerous errors into which Galen had unavoidably fallen. The awe and reverence for the name of Galen was so great that his statement regarding the rupture of the peritoneum in hernia was generally accepted up to the time of [the Swiss doctor Albrecht von] Haller (1708-1777)."

A hernia is a gradual stretching of the tissues and escape of the abdominal contents either into a preformed or congenital sac or, as in the common acquired type, by the formation of a sac from the peritoneal lining of the abdomen. Abdominal herniae are named from the part through which they pass, as inguinal, femoral or umbilical. The scrotal or labial herniae are simply the inguinal herniae so developed that the sac and its contents has emerged from the external abdominal ring and entered the scrotum or labia. We may also find the ventral hernia: a protrusion through any part of the anterior abdominal wall except at the unbilicus or above it; the epigastric hernia: a protrusion of peritoneum in the space bounded by the ensiform cartilage, the ribs and the umbilicus; the obturator hernia: a protrusion through the obturator membrane or obturator canal, and felt below the horizontal ramus of the pubes internal to the femoral vessels.

. . . Causes of Hernia. It is most liable to occur in the male. It occurs at any period of life and sometimes hereditary predisposition seems to exist. Sometimes a mass of fat forms in the canal before the hernia appears and it seems to have a causative relation to it. Any strenuous occupation predisposes to hernia. Weak, flabby abdominal muscles, predispose to hernia. Muscular relaxation from ill-health, or following pregnancy, and wounds or scars following operations, or abscesses may predispose to hernia. The exciting causes are muscular effort, lifting, strains, jumping, sudden effort to guard in falling, and so on.

When a hernia is forming the person feels a muscular pain in the lower abdomen, which is intensified on sneezing or coughing. This may be noticed weeks before it is evident that a hernia is present. If a hernia is suspected, careful examination should be made. Insert the tip of the little finger in the external ring and ask the patient to cough. Where a hernia is present, succession will be detected on coughing. In a healthy person no more than the tip of the little finger can be inserted in the external ring. If the top of the index finger can be inserted the aperture is dilated and even if there is no hernia present one may safely be prognosed. In examining the external ring in a man, invert the skin of the scrotum and carry the finger into the ring.

Reducible Hernia. In reducing a hernia, no instrument surpasses the human hand. When a hernia is reducible the contents of the sac can be emptied into the abdominal cavity. But unless the sac can be reduced with the contents out of the inguinal canal into the abdominal cavity, the case is surgical and requires radical treatment. *Most cases are curable by exercise before the sac is adhered* [my emphasis, L.S.]. **After the sac is adhered it requires long continued proper use of the abdominal muscles to produce the desired results.** *Correct use of any muscle tends to make it normal* [my emphasis, L.S.].

The shape of the sac can be felt in the reducible hernia. There is a smooth enlargement at a known hernial opening, larger below than above, which began above and extended downward. It is often possible to feel the neck. In enterocele the enlargement becomes smaller and may disappear altogether on lying down. Straining, lifting, or standing, especially while leaning forward, makes the mass more prominent; cough causes impulse or succussion [violent shaking]. The protrusion is elastic and there is a gurgling sound when the mass suddenly disappears on reduction. In epiplocele the mass is less elastic. It is often irregular and compressible and feels doughy. There is little impulse on coughing, and muscular effort or standing has little influence on its size. Percussion gives a dull note and reduction is accomplished slowly and no gurgling sound results.[91]

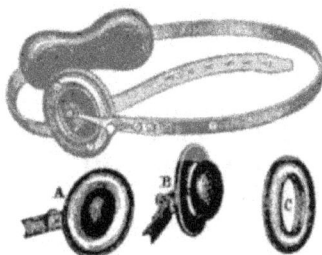

Victorian hard rubber truss, designed to make both general and concentrated pressure. A) ring with center pad; B) center pad projected from ring; C) ring alone.

MOST HERNIAS ARE GENETICALLY INHERITED
Although a hernia can indeed occur from "violent muscular exertions" alone (such as lifting heavy objects), according to medical authorities this is rare compared to the actual number one cause: a "weakness and laxity of the peritoneum, together with a general laxity in the abdominal muscles."[92] Some believe that this "weakness and laxity" is almost always a "hereditary predisposition," giving rise to what are labeled "hernial families": disease-affected fathers and mothers who pass their hernial genes onto their children, and so on, *ad infinitum.*[93]

On this interesting topic Dr. Albert John Ochsner and Nelson M. Percy write in their 1912 book *A New Clinical Surgery*:

☛ **There can be no doubt but that there is an hereditary tendency in many families to the formation of hernia. If** both parents in a family suffer from this defect some of the children are almost certain to be afflicted in the same manner. The well-known fact that special defects in families are likely to be inherited is shown in this disease. [For example:] There is a much larger proportion of herniae in nationalities in which intermarriage between first cousins is freely practised than in others in which this is forbidden.[94]

In a 1925 essay, "The Inguinal Hernia," which appeared in the *Journal of the Missouri State Medical Association*, Dr. Ross A. Woolsey states that:

☞ Hernia is the sequel of a congenital defect often made apparent by effort. Its protrusion through the abdominal wall is quite gradual and has existed there for a long time, easily recognized by one accustomed to such examinations.[95]

In his 1876 book *The Principles and Practice of Surgery*, Dr. Frank Hastings Hamilton writes similarly of congenital inguinal hernia in males:

☞ The term "congenital," as applied to this form of hernia, does not imply that the visceral protrusion exists at birth; but only that the peculiar anatomical condition exists, dating from and anterior to the period of birth, which favors its occurrence. In many cases the viscera do not escape until adult life, and in nearly all cases the protrusion takes place subsequent to birth, usually within the first few weeks or months.[96]

HERNIAS & INDUSTRIAL WORK
Inevitably such views led to the notion that "every man who develops this condition [a hernia], was born with potential hernia."[97] In other words, proponents of this theory hold that the hernial sac is almost always congenital and that the adult hernia is merely "the enlargement of a congenital hernia later in life."[98]

Evidence for this view derives from the railroad industry. In 1919 Dr. C. W. Hopkins writes:

☞ No doubt there are cases of true traumatic hernia, but in railroad surgery in particular, which calls for the care of patients who have received severe falls or squeezings through the abdomen and pelvis, causing most extreme intra-abdominal pressure, sufficient to cause rupture of the bladder, kidney, liver, intestines, or to crush the pelvis, why is it that inguinal hernia is never found as a concomitant unless the injuries were probably of sufficient severity to cause death?

Taking into consideration the fact that there are thousands of men of all ages who are engaged every day in occupations requiring heavy lifting, hard straining, or are engaged in acrobatic work, which frequently calls for the most strenuous effort and muscular action, particularly of the abdominal muscles, and who sustain severe falls, if extraordinary muscular effort or great intra-abdominal pressure are the chief causes of hernia, why are not all of these men victims of hernia?[99]

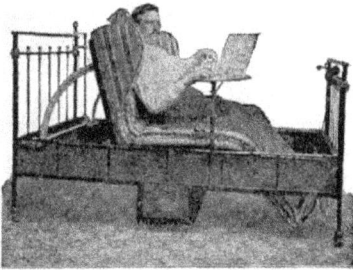

Adjustable beds, like this Victorian model from the late 1800s, were often used by individuals suffering from the debilitating disease known as inguinal hernia.

Whether from genetics or trauma, the fact remains the same: most inguinal hernias are not caused by some form of physical violence to the body, and are therefore not actual "ruptures" or "rips" in the muscular tissue. Rather, a majority are the slow and gradual product (sometimes lifelong) of genetically predisposed feeble and infirm abdominal muscles through which the viscera find a natural opening to protrude from.

In his 1915 article "Traumatic Hernia, and its Relation to the Workmen's Compensation Act," Dr. R. Robinson Duff writes:

☛ Real traumatic hernia is an injury to the abdominal (belly) wall of sufficient severity to puncture or tear asunder said wall, and permit the exposure or protruding of the abdominal viscera or some part thereof. Such an injury will be compensated. . . . All other hernias, whenever occurring or discovered, and whatsoever the cause . . . are considered to be diseases causing incapacitating conditions or permanent partial disability.

But the permanent partial disability and the causes of such are considered to be as shown by medical facts—to have either existed from birth; to have been years in formation and duration, or both, and are not compensatory. . . .[100]

TRUE TRAUMATIC HERNIAS ARE RARE

Traumatic hernias are so rare, some physicians believe they do not exist. Writing in 1902, Dr. Hobart Amory Hare notes the following:

☛ In referring to the attitude of the profession generally toward the question of traumatic hernia, Bilfinger cites the opinions of Roser, König, Socin, and others, all to the effect that the sudden development of a hernial sac is impossible, or at least incompatible, with their experiences.

The number of those who admit the possibility of the occurrence of a hernia on a purely traumatic basis, as a result of trauma, is small. Witzel believes that through undue stretching or bending of the body backward, etc., fissures may be produced in the linea alba through which, either immediately or some time after the injury, a small hernia may extrude. Orth and Seidel, too, have acknowledged the traumatic origin of these herniæ. Streubel admits that traumatic hernia do occur in direct connection with subcutaneous muscular ruptures.

Graser states: "It is the consensus of opinion among those who have given the subject most careful attention that the sudden complete development of a hernia is a very rare occurrence—so rare that it is hardly of any significance from a practical stand-point."[101]

The reason for the fact that nearly all surgeons deny the existence of traumatic herniæ, Bilfinger states, is to be found, partially, in the uncertainty of intra-abdominal pressure; partially, in the theoretical impossibility of an explanation, and, lastly, in the unsuccessful experiments.

Bilfinger describes the experiments that have been made in order to throw light upon the question of traumatic hernia, and states that while it has been impossible so far to produce traumatic hernia by experiment, it must be considered that a number of conditions come into play which it is difficult to produce artificially, and these support one another in a very definite way in the individual case. He adds that, while the negative results of the experiments support the view that traumatic hernia are rare, the mechanism must be very complicated; they do not speak against traumatic hernia.[102]

Here is more evidence, if more be needed, that if you have an inguinal hernia it is almost certainly the result of a congenital disease, namely, genetically inherited feeble abdominal musculature.[103]

YOUR INGUINAL HERNIA IS MOST LIKELY A DISEASE
This fact was so well-known *and* accepted during the Victorian Period that it was taken for granted. And indeed, countless 19th-Century surgeons reported that the number one cause of inguinal hernias was not a "tear" in the abdominal lining, but a weak abdominal area—one that "can be cured by strengthening." In his 1880 *A Practical Treatise on Hernia* Joseph H. Warren writes:

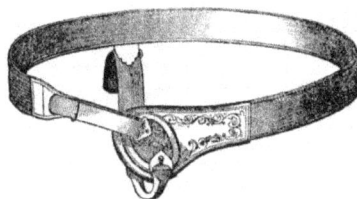

Victorian elastic truss, with perineal band.

☞ . . . we find hernia most common, not in subjects who have elongated mesenteries [a continuous double folded band of tissue or membrane that attaches to the wall of the abdomen and encloses the organs], but in those in whom the abdominal parietes [walls] are deficient or insufficient, and that it is an indisputable fact that *hernias have been cured by strengthening these containing parietes* [my emphasis, L.S.]. If hernia were primarily and principally due to an abnormal elongation of the mesentery, any attempt to cure it, by occluding the opening and strengthening the wall, must be either useless or result in a protrusion in some other weakened part.[104]

Warren then goes on to discuss the "predisposing causes of hernia." These include:

☞ Whatever tends to diminish the resistance of the abdominal walls, such as a weakened constitution, laxity of the fibrous tissues, congenital enlargement of the canal, ascites, pregnancy, old age, etc. Poverty and hard work thus favor the production of hernia. Men, who have larger abdominal rings than women, are the more liable to inguinal hernia; while women who have a deeper and wider femoral arch than men, and usually smaller muscles over the space, are relatively more subject to femoral hernia. [Also, whatever] . . . increases the volume, weight, or mobility of the contained parts; such as hypertrophy of the viscera from whatever cause, deposition of fat in the omentum, etc.

. . . [Another cause of hernia is the] gradual expulsion of the parietal peritoneal membrane at weak parts of the abdominal walls. This protrusion is produced by whatever calls into play the violent simultaneous action of the diaphragm and the abdominal muscles. This action, which constitutes the act of straining, plays an important part in the production of hernia, even when the containing parietes possess their usual strength. It is most strikingly exemplified in lifting heavy weights, leaping, singing, especially in deep tones, and in playing on wind instruments; in the powerful and irregular acts of excessive coition, vomiting, coughing, horseback riding, and some military exercises; in certain diseases, as calculus, constipation, asthma; in excessive exertions immediately after a full meal, or during the state of pregnancy, in the exertions attending difficult parturition, and in the forcible attempts to evacuate the rectum or bladder made by persons afflicted with stricture, enlarged prostrate, stone in the bladder, and constipation.[105]

Dr. Tillmanns provided the following details on the etiology or cause of hernias in 1898:

☛ There have been various theories regarding the etiology of herniæ. In congenital herniæ we have primarily to do with a malformation or abnormality in the development of the involved part of the abdominal wall. In acquired herniæ various factors have to be considered. The intra-abdominal pressure exerted upon parts of the abdominal wall which are less capable of resistance plays an especially important part. . . . [It has been observed that] **when treating of the various forms of herniæ . . . certain parts of the abdominal wall, in consequence of their diminished resistance, are predisposed to the development of hernia. The following conditions are also of importance in connection with their development: Abnormal length and relaxation of the mesentery, as well as a low position of its insertion; and, finally, abundant fat in the subperitoneal cellular tissue of the parietal peritoneum, which by its growth externally drags the peritonæum after it in the form of a pouch. This outward traction, caused by subperitoneal lipomata, is probably a rare factor. The anatomical character of certain parts of the abdominal wall is of great importance in the origin of a hernia, especially**

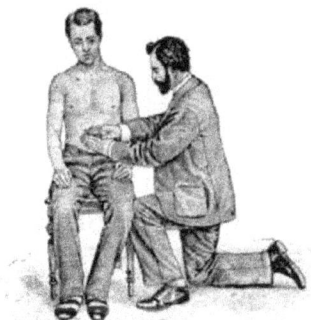

Victorian doctor diagnosing an inguinal hernia.

normal or abnormal openings—e.g., the inguinal and the femoral canals; also defective closure of the peritoneal cavity, a diminished resistance of the abdominal wall, and cicatrices after wounds, after operations, etc. In addition to this anatomical predisposition, there is an exciting cause which sometimes acts suddenly and sometimes gradually in the production of a hernia. We seek this determining cause chiefly in the greater or less increase of intra-abdominal pressure—e.g., from the constant lifting of heavy burdens, from frequent coughing, singing, screaming, blowing, or pressing, or in connection with chronic constipation, etc. Hernia is accordingly to some extent an occupation disease. The parietal peritonæum yields more and more to the increased intra-abdominal pressure at the weak place in the abdominal wall, and a protrusion is formed here, into which the viscera gradually pass. In some cases the abdominal viscera are forced suddenly into a preformed hernial sac, under the influence of an exciting cause. In other cases displacement of the abdominal organs occurs suddenly from an injury of the abdominal wall or from a rent in the peritoneum or the

diaphragm. *These traumatic herniæ are not true herniæ, inasmuch as they possess no hernial sac. The hernial sac—that is, the true hernia—is always developed gradually, though an injury may, of course, act the part of the exciting cause* [my emphasis, L.S.]. The supposed sudden development of a true hernia is, in my opinion, always dependent upon a mistake in observation. The hernial sac, as a rule, is already present, but is empty, or the hernia already formed at the time of the injury was so small as not to have been noticed. I therefore agree with Socin that a hernia, from the medico-legal point of view, is not to be designated exclusively as an "injury." The herniæ supposed to have arisen "suddenly in consequence of an injury" are in part a result of the traumatism, but are due in part to a special condition of the body of the injured person which already existed.[106]

CONGENITAL HERNIA VS. TRAUMATIC HERNIA
In the 1921 book *Surgical Diagnosis and Treatment*, Dr. E. Wyllys Andrews writes of the medical confusion surrounding congenital hernias and traumatic hernias:

☛ Much discussion has occurred on the problem of trauma as opposed to congenital defect in the causation of hernia. This has been made a subject of controversy in connection with problems of accident insurance and personal injury suits for damages. Many pathologists take the ground that all hernias are of congenital origin. To support this view it can be shown that the affection is markedly hereditary, that a large number of adults who acquire hernias are found to have had the same affection in childhood, and that upon operation a great proportion of them prove to have the congenital preformed sac which clearly brought on the condition. On the other hand, trauma, when it can be proved, is usually found to have been some minor injury, as in lifting, or some unimportant strain. Perhaps it is too much to assert that traumatic hernia apart from congenital defect never is produced in the inguinal or femoral region, but very few cases can be discovered in which the history of injury is unmixed in this respect.[107]

In 1919 Dr. Lauffer gave this explanation of how a congenital or acquired hernia may form:

☛ **The dimple of the peritoneum at the internal ring may deepen, and extend along the perivascular spaces; or the protrusion of peritoneum may arise owing to weak fascial and deficient muscular support. (The direct inguinal hernia results from relaxed fascial support.) The acquired hernial sac arises slowly, because the peritoneum is a tough, resistant membrane, and cannot be pushed out to form a sac by any single impulse. This is readily demonstrated on the cadaver; no finger is strong enough to push out the peritoneum suddenly at the internal ring. Yet *nature permits the gradual stretching of the peritoneum without tearing it* [my emphasis, L.S.], as in the acquired type of hernial sacs.**[108]

Dr. Lauffer strictly differentiates an acquired hernia from a traumatic hernia, the former which is generally caused by weak or flabby abdominal tissues, and the latter, which is the result of a violent exertion of or on the body:

☛ *The traumatic hernia:* . . . **A traumatic abdominal hernia is not confined to the hernial zones, but may arise wherever sufficient external violence is applied.** *In the truly traumatic hernia, the peritoneum is torn; there is no sac, the viscera came out through a fresh tear in the peritoneum* [my emphasis, L.S.]. **Direct injury, such as might be caused by the horn of a mad bull, or by the tongue of a wagon drawn by runaway horses, inflicting sufficient violence to the physical structures of the body, may produce traumatic hernia at the site of the focal trauma.**
Falls from high structures often cause multiple fractures, and ruptures of internal organs, but seldom give rise to traumatic hernia. A violent squeeze, such as occurs when a railroader is caught between a moving car and a station platform, it is stated, may so increase intra-abdominal pressure, as to tear the peritoneum and cause a true traumatic hernia. *So infrequent is traumatic hernia, however, that many industrial surgeons of wide experience have never encountered one* [my emphasis, L.S.].[109]

It is for these very reasons that the acquired (reducible inguinal) hernia, which forms the vast majority of hernia types, is considered by nearly all physicians to be a "disease," while the much rarer traumatic hernia is classified as an "injury." In other words, most if not all acquired hernias seem to derive from a congenital weakness of the abdominal tissues, a type of hernia that, both experience and science have proven, can often be repaired or cured naturally at home without surgery.[110] It is the traumatic hernia—a sac-less tear in the abdominal tissues—which usually requires surgery. Thus, Dr. Charles H. May writes in 1919:

☛ **I believe . . . that there is an anatomical defect in the individual who develops inguinal hernia following straining or accident—that he has a congenital protrusion of the sac along the cord. A true traumatic hernia, if inguinal, is nearly as much of an injury as if it were produced on the abdomen in other regions. It should be accompanied by such local evidence of its occurrence [e.g., bruising, cuts, swelling, scrapes, blood, etc.] as would be expected from injury of the parts.[111]**

JOB RELATED HERNIAS ARE UNCOMMON

Despite the clear demarcation between acquired and traumatic inguinal hernias, the two continue to be confused with one another. This has resulted in, for example, millions of dollars a year in compensation being wrongfully awarded to workers whose hernias

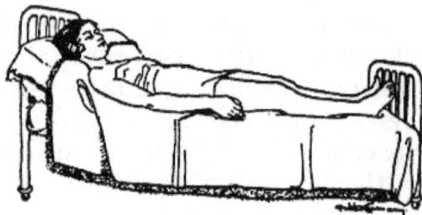

Bed rest is often required for inguinal hernia.

were not the result of an "injury" on the job, but instead were the product of an incipient or congenital disease—that is, genetically weak abdominal tissue. This condition (disease), of course, is not covered by workman's compensation. Only authentic traumatic hernias would meet this requirement. Thus, in the case of industrial accidents, medical jurisprudence now requires that:

☛ **A hernia, in order to be entitled to an indemnity, must be of recent origin, it must appear suddenly, must be accompanied by pain, and must immediately follow an accident. There must be proof that the hernia did not exist prior to the accident.[112]**

THE DISEASE KNOWN AS INGUINAL HERNIA
The knowledge that a hernia is, in fact, not usually the result of an accident but rather a disease has been known for at least a century or more. In the 1908 book *Surgery: Its Principles and Practice*, Dr. William B. Coley writes:

☛ [When applied specifically to the abdominal area] **the term hernia has come to be synonymous with rupture, and is applied to a protrusion of some one or more of the abdominal viscera, through a normal or an abnormal opening. While rupture is the term most commonly used by the laity in describing this condition, it is misleading, since it rests upon a false conception of the etiology. The term originated at a time when it was generally believed that traumatism, or tearing of the muscular structures by some direct or indirect violence, was a frequent and important cause. The great increase in our knowledge, as a result of the large number of operations for the radical cure of hernia that have been performed during the last two decades, has proved that** *in the vast majority of cases "hernia is a disease rather than an accident." In other words, it is due to a congenital defect, e.g., an open funicular process of peritoneum, or an abnormal size of some normal opening in the abdominal wall. This congenital defect, then, is the main cause of a hernia, while the immediate or exciting cause plays but a minor role* [my emphasis, L.S.].[113]

HOW TO DISTINGUISH CONGENITAL & TRAUMATIC
It being true that nearly all hernias result from disease and only a small almost negligible minority actually derive from injury, the question naturally arises: Is it possible to tell the two apart? Dr. Coley answers the inquiry this way:

☛ **It may sometimes be possible to distinguish a congenital or preformed sac from an actually acquired hernial sac, i.e., one formed after birth, by the intimacy of its relationship to the cord and its vessels in the male, and to the round ligament in the female. The acquired sac, a type of which we have in the direct hernia, is simply a bulging forward of the parietal peritoneum into some opening or weak place in the abdominal wall. This sac has no intimate connection with the cord or the round ligament.**

In a preformed or congenital sac, on the other hand, we find, especially in children (and this is equally true whether the sac connects with the tunica vaginalis or not), the sac in the most intimate relationship with the cord and cord vessels, the latter lying in closest contact with the thin membrane of the sac, and both surrounded by the infundibuliform fascia. In many cases the sac extends down to the tunica vaginalis testis without communicating with it. But such communication is of no importance in estimating its claim to being classed as congenital. *Some writers have recently gone so far as to class all inguinal and femoral hernias as congenital* [my emphasis, L.S.], with the possible exception of some cases of direct inguinal hernia. This position has been taken and most ably defended by R. Hamilton Russell, of Melbourne. Russell has seen a direct hernial sac in the cadaver of a man who had no hernia during life. A number of similar cases of congenital pouches of peritoneum have been found in the femoral region, in which cases there was no history of hernia during life. Furthermore, Russell cites much evidence based on embryologic research, which seems to prove that such pouches of peritoneum actually do occur, and not infrequently in the femoral canal. Whether these be regarded as a normal event of "developmental accident" is of no particular moment. If these facts be true, we have a better explanation of the origin of femoral hernia than any that has hitherto been offered.[114]

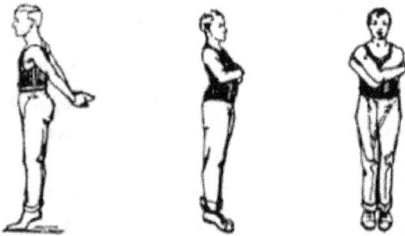

As we shall see shortly, exercise and physical fitness are key to self-treating inguinal hernia.

THE GOOD NEWS FOR INGUINAL HERNIA SUFFERERS
I have included this somewhat detailed medical information here because it is good news for the average hernia sufferer. Why? It shows that the vast majority of inguinal hernias in adults are *acquired*, and are the result of a congenital *disease*, a genetically inherited "defect" that causes an abnormal stretching or widening of the natural openings in the abdominal tissues. This makes an

acquired hernia highly amenable to natural self-healing therapies, as well as much less likely to need surgery. On the other hand, the quite uncommon *traumatic* hernia is the result of an *injury*, which forms an actual "rip" in the fabric of the abdominal tissues. This makes it less susceptible to home-treatment because it must *always* require surgery to mend it.

If you have an inguinal hernia then, it is probably acquired, making you a potential candidate for natural treatment. Your doctor will be able to help you determine what kind of hernia you have; and, whether or not it is an acquired (i.e., congenital) one, or a traumatic (i.e., injurious) one, and whether or not you qualify for a non-surgical, self-therapeutic program like those presented by Victorian doctors and myself in this book. In either case you must always be diagnosed by a qualified physician before embarking on any home remedial plan.

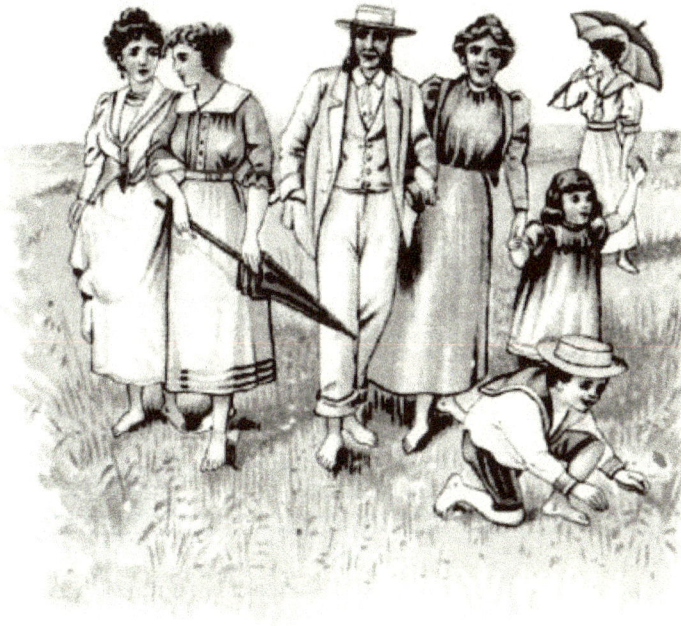

During the Victorian Era walking barefoot in wet grass was a common contributing remedy for all types of ailments, including inguinal hernia.

Ad for a 1923 Vegetarian Cook Book

The Victorian author of the above book, Dr. Henry Lindlahr, prescribed a vegetarian diet to those suffering from, among many other maladies, inguinal hernia. In the author's opinion, however, it is questionable whether a vegetarian diet could ever fulfil the requirements needed to heal a hernia, which necessitates elevated levels of protein and vitamin D, both difficult to procure without consuming animal products—namely, meat, dairy, and eggs.

3

Victorian Home Treatments for Inguinal Hernia

TWO OF THE MOST HARMFUL HERNIA MYTHS

Today's hernia sufferers are fortunate indeed to live in the 21st Century. In his 1852 book *Permanent Cure of Reducible Hernia*, Dr. George Hayward writes that:

☞ **Cauterization, ligature, sutures, excision . . . and castration were the principal operative** [hernia cure] **methods in use for eighteen hundred years. The object of all of them was to . . . prevent the protrusion of any of the abdominal contents.**[15]

Along with vast improvements in treatment, modern naturopathic medicine is debunking numerous old myths associated with inguinal hernias, the two most pernicious being that: 1) hernias cannot be cured in the elderly or even in the middle aged (only in children), and that, 2) hernias more than 6-12 months old will not respond to natural or nonsurgical treatment. Both of these notions are patently false.

In fact, as we shall see, Victorian hernia doctors routinely and successfully

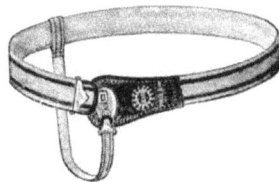

An ordinary Victorian elastic truss.

treated both adults and elderly patients,[116] as well as individuals of all ages, with hernias more than a decade old.[117] One 19th-Century clinic, for example, destroyed both fictions simultaneously by curing a 78 year old man with a 15 year old inguinal hernia in just three months—*"without any surgical operation, pain, or suspension of the patient's ordinary avocations."*[118] In 1821 Dufour promises that the medical establishment will

☛ . . . soon learn by proofs the most irrefragable, that . . . [hernia] cures, with scarcely an exception, take place in adults; and as to "old subjects," . . . [conventional doctors] will also be apprized that [hernia] cures bear the same wonderful proportion; for even as to them . . . every thing may be believed and expected, but failure in the means adopted by us to effect cure.[119]

ROOTS OF THE INGUINAL HERNIA CURE
Having ascertained the basic cause of this hereditary disease—in full properly called an *adult, congenital, incomplete, reducible, inguinal hernia*—we are now prepared to study its treatments, for as Dr. Arnaud stated in 1748:

☛ It is an established principle, that by destroying the causes of diseases, the effects of them must cease of course.[120]

In 1878 Dr. Hayes Agnew gave the following advice on treating hernias, dividing the remedies into two categories, "palliative" and "radical":

☛ The treatment of hernia is divided into the palliative and the radical. The palliative method consists in restoring the hernial contents to the cavity of the abdomen, and retaining them there by a properly-fitting truss. This should be done at the earliest possible moment. No patient is safe so long as the rupture remains outside of the body. Children form no exception to this rule . . .[121]

Note: As his use of the word palliative (meaning, treating symptoms only) attests, Dr. Agnew was one of a number of Victorian medical professionals who did not believe that a hernia could be cured without resorting to surgery, a erroneous belief that has been thoroughly disproven since his day—as my own natural, non-surgical healing experience, and that of thousands of others, aptly demonstrates.

EXERCISES THAT AID IN INGUINAL HERNIA HEALING
During the Victorian Era, arguably the number one component of *naturally* healing a reducible inguinal hernia was what were then called "curative gymnastics" or "room gymnastics": physical exercises designed to develop strength and coordination while building up the immune system and overall health. This is still the primary method of self-treating an inguinal hernia, though today we would call this method *anaerobic exercise* (short bursts of physical exertion), defined as general strength training via such activities as *brief* sessions of weight lifting, circuit training, planks, Pilates, yoga, lunges, pushups, squats, burpees, jumping rope, sprints, pull-ups, and sit-ups.[122]

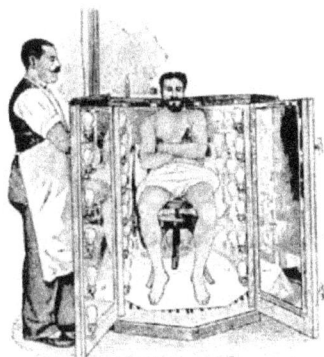

Victorian doctors sometimes turned to light therapy to aid in healing. This gentleman is taking an electric light bath at the Bilz Sanatorium in Germany, circa 1898.

Though this book focuses mainly on anaerobic exercises, before we go any further it is important to mention here that *aerobic exercise* (sustained physical exertion) can also greatly benefit the hernia sufferer. This is defined as general health development via such activities as *extended* sessions of walking, swimming, hiking, skipping, rowing, bike riding, treadmilling, jumping jacks, dancing, climbing, skiing, and jogging.[123]

THE BILZ PROGRAM: INTRODUCTION
The Victorian health practitioner had much to say on both curative gymnastics and preparing for a session of curative gymnastics. In 1898 Friedrich Eduard Bilz wrote the following (to be done with an assistant):

☞ . . . in a normal condition the walls of the so called passage [that is, the inguinal canal] touch each other closely, remaining however elastic and serving as a natural protection to the tissues, ligaments and spermatic cords,

and thus prevent a rupture [i.e., an abnormal widening, relaxation, or stretching of the opening] **taking place by supporting and strengthening the inner and outer tissues.** *The only means of obviating a relaxation and closing the orifice of the hernial sacks in case of rupture having taken place, is by strengthening the tissues in question* [my emphasis, L.S.]. **This is done by massage of the abdomen and the region of the rupture and by** *appropriate curative gymnastics, especially by resistance exercises of the legs and trunk* [my emphasis, L.S.] **and for their support other Modes of Application of the Natural Method whereby not only the whole of the abdominal walls but also the whole of the intestines (bowels and the internal organs of the abdomen) are strengthened. This cure must be** [i.e., will be] **a thorough** [one], **and not only in new and light cases but also in old and obstinate ones.**

The patient must, until the tissues in question have become stronger, wear a well fitting truss, that is this truss must fit in such a manner (especially during gymnastics, etc.) that it will not form impediment to free movement. Therefore it is advisable that the patient should have a truss fitting closely, while the body is at ease, and one fitting loosely while performing the exercises. It is well to sound the place occasionally when the hernia is located with the fingers so as to ascertain whether during violent movements the rupture [i.e., an abnormally enlarged opening as opposed to a tear] **shows a tendency to protrude or remains in the recess of the abdomen.**

As soon as the treatment shows satisfactory results the truss may now and again be removed (during the gymnastic exercises only conditionally) and gradually be left off all together. During the process of massage and the performance of gymnastic exercises it is of vital importance that the abdominal wall be in a relaxed state, therefore deep breathing is recommended.

All the movements during the exercises must be executed towards the seat of the rupture (not away from it): it is moreover to be strictly kept in view, that the massage and all movements during the exercises are done slowly, not too vigorously or too frequently. Should dislocations occur in other parts of the abdomen, a thing which rarely occurs, the same treatment is applicable.

THE BILZ PROGRAM: TREATMENT

First of all rub the affected part with the tips of your fingers, which may be dry or wet, with a circular movement several times a day for the space of from one to five minutes: then have the abdomen massaged (kneading, pressing and beating it), [after which] further introduce the active passive and resistance movements of the trunk and legs towards the seat of the rupture; then lift the body from a lying position into a sitting one and move slowly back again on the side of the rupture.

In the same position, after the leg has been moved a little sidewards from the other one, the patient should, the masseur slightly resisting it, move this leg back again to close with the other one, repeating this in both directions, but with the pressure always towards the seat of the hernia.

After this each leg (the one on the side of the ruptured part more frequently) should be lifted towards the body, then both legs together with resistance on the part of the attendant, do this with the legs stretched and bent, then lower them slack. The same procedure is to be observed with the back supported and in a sitting position with the legs hanging down, hereafter the knees should be drawn up and spread and then closed, the attendant resisting, the same to be done with the legs stretched out. The spreading is to be done with the legs slack, the closing vigorously.

In support of these exercises one to two hip-baths a day at a temperature of 77°F to 86°F and lasting from five to ten minutes should be taken, including a kneading of the abdomen. Furthermore apply water to the rupture by means of a squirt or by pouring it from a vessel held in an elevated position. As a further expedient a small wet cloth is to be worn under the truss renewing and cleansing it from time to time.[124]

As we shall see in the next section, like many Victorian physicians, Dr. Bilz recommended gymnastics: various short but vigorous bouts of exercise. This idea—that any improvement in one's total health will also expedite the healing of an inguinal hernia—is a sound one, and is as true and useful today as it was 125 years ago.

THE BILZ PROGRAM: GYMNASTICS

☞ Remarks on gymnastics at home: also called active, as distinguished from passive, movements of the muscles.

Our entire organic life depends on the process of assimilation, which can only be maintained in a normal state by the exercise of every part of the body. The more we stimulate this process by bodily exercise the more will our life gain in freshness, strength, and endurance; and the better we shall be able to ward off bad health and disease, and to overcome them if they attack us.

If the process of assimilation is imperfect—in other words, where there exists congestion of blood and of the substances of the body, a state of things usually resulting when there is in sufficient bodily exercise—our first task must be to further the assimilating process in the whole system—or, as the case may be, in single parts of the body—and to restore it to its normal condition; in order to bring about the excretion of morbid refuse matter, which has remained behind in the system, and to give new energy to all the organs of the body. In the attainment of this end curative gymnastics play an important part; because they incite the various muscles to general and many-sided activity, the want of which results in obstruction of the process of assimilation—in a word, in ill health.

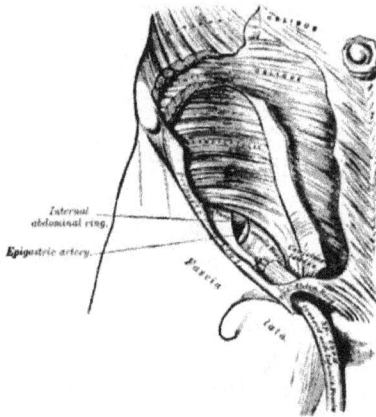

Dissection of an inguinal hernia, showing the transversalis muscle, the transversalis fascia, and the internal abdominal ring. The navel is in the upper right.

Another fruitful source of ill health is the neglect of vigorous respiration, which is the natural consequence of insufficient bodily exercise. It is only by deep breathing that good and richly oxygenated blood can be formed. A person, therefore, who is obliged to spend his time sitting or standing, should not neglect to practise regular gymnastic exercises.

Too much sitting, which fails to give the abdominal muscles the opportunity of exercising their functions, leads to disturbance of digestion, gastric weakness, constipation, defective formation of blood, congestion of the liver and spleen (the whole system belonging to the portal vein) the consequences of which are, in their turn, chlorosis, anæmia, nervousness, chronic headache, vertigo, hypochondria, hysteria, melancholy, scrofula, etc.

Although the disadvantages of insufficient bodily exercise may not be apparent during the prime of life, the evil consequences are sure to be felt in after years. We are then threatened with a whole host of chronic complaints, such as piles, gout, asthma, congestion, abdominal complaints, paralysis, hysteria, hypochondria, melancholia, fluor albus; as well as the diseases named in the foregoing paragraph, and besides stiff limbs and bodily deformity.

It need hardly be mentioned that it is absolutely necessary that attention to the skin should go hand in hand with gymnastic exercises of every kind, if we would guard against illness.

How many thousands of ladies there are in the higher grades of society who, without being perhaps seriously ill, are nearly always ailing and out of health; and who would be well if they were to take regular exercise, practise curative gymnastics every day, and pay proper attention to the skin.

Curative gymnastics, also called room gymnastics, are of special value because they may be easily performed anywhere—in the room before an open window, in the garden, or during a walk in some sequestered spot, or while travelling—and because they need no assistance from other persons.

By the practice of curative gymnastics, not only are diseases warded off, or has been mentioned, but they can be cured, as the name "curative gymnastics" implies [my emphasis, L.S.]. **The principles and methods upon and by which the gymnastics should be applied in various diseases, are indicated in a general manner in the articles treating of the diseases** [not included in this book, L.S.].[125] **In the first place I would draw attention to the following observations on curative gymnastics.**

THE BILZ PROGRAM: REMARKS ON CURATIVE EXERCISE

1. Be it expressly observed that, in the application of curative gymnastics, as in any other treatment, it is of vital importance that the means employed should exactly correspond with the circumstances of each individual case, (i.e., in treating a patient, regard must be had to the existing reserve of vital force). This, however, can only be judged by a professional man [or woman].

2. The gymnastics must not be applied in serious cases, where inflammatory and feverish conditions exist; nor should pregnant persons have recourse to any exhaustive form of curative gymnastics, but they should restrict themselves to very gentle movements, such as taking walks, etc. *Patients suffering from abdominal hernia must take great care, when practising movements which bring the abdominal muscles into play, that their truss keeps the hernia completely under control* [my emphasis, L.S.].

3. The movements must be executed calmly and without hurry; but energetically, and with full exertion of the muscles; as much as possible in accordance with the illustration and description given; if they cannot all be successfully performed at once they will by practice become easy of accomplishment. If, however, by reason of some physical peculiarity, the patient is unable to perform a movement, let him omit it for the time, rather than make violent efforts to perform it. The body may by practice become capable of performing it with ease: it is surprising, indeed, what progress even elderly persons can make in this respect.

4. It is advisable always to take the easier exercises in hand first, and by degrees to advance to the more difficult ones. We must here remind the reader, once more, always to adapt the duration and number of the different exercises to his strength and bodily condition. He may always consider the feeling of fatigue or pain as an indication that it is time to stop; and that hint must never be disregarded. Two things must be kept in view in connection with these exercises: (a) the patient must feel completely rested, before going on again with a fresh exercise; and (b) there should be no sharp muscular pain after the completion of the practice. Beginners, in particular, should never lose sight of these two conditions: if, notwithstanding the greatest prudence and

the gentlest movements, considerable muscular pain makes its appearance, a pause must be made until the pain has subsided; and then some quite gentle and easy exercise only should be taken.

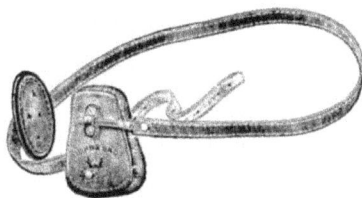

An Army and Navy truss during the Victorian Period.

5. Although a patient's performance may be very poor at first, he will be able in a short time, as soon as he is used to the movements, to perform double and three times as much, and more; and to stand it better than when he began. Should the exercises even cause him some trouble and pain at the outset, he must not at once run away with the idea that he cannot master them, or that they are beyond his strength; but he must quietly continue with them, always having regard to the limits imposed by his constitutional powers.

6. The best time to perform the exercises is from a quarter of an hour to half an hour before a meal. It is well to associate them with the daily meals; if for no other reason than that we may have something to remind us of our practise; for the first conditions of success are regularity and perseverance. It is advisable, therefore, that arrangements be made to practise the exercises every day a short time before breakfast or dinner. If the evening be fixed for them, the time chosen should be about a couple of hours before going to bed.

7. Previously to beginning the exercises, all tight clothing must be removed from neck, chest and abdomen.

8. During the intervals of rest, of which there should be several whilst going through a group of exercises, the patient should endeavour to breathe deeply, calmly, fully and strongly; in doing which he places his hands on his hips, or against the back of his head, and takes care to empty the lungs thoroughly at every respiration. In each of the gymnastic exercises the moment should be noted when a deep breath becomes necessary; and breath should be taken at that point in each repetition of the exercise. When a pause for breathing exercises is made between the groups of gymnastic movements, or after

each single exercise, six or eight deep respirations should be taken. Such breathing exercises should never be omitted; and may well be taken after every two gymnastic movements.

9. The motto in this, as in any other curative treatment, should be "Don't overdo it." We must not imagine that our gain will be in proportion to the number of exercises gone through. We really gain in health when and so long only as improvement in the nutrition of the body—i.e., the renewal of used-up organic substances—keeps pace with the muscular movements. So long as this balance is maintained, increased vital power and energy will result from the practice of gymnastics: but if they are carried too far, the result will be the opposite of that intended; namely, increased weakness and exhaustion. On well-selected exercises and a moderate use of them, therefore, a sure and favourable result depends; and this can only be attained by degrees.

10. If breathing and pulsation have been sensibly accelerated by any given exercise, we must wait till they are quiet again before proceeding to the next movement.

11. After the muscular strength has been gradually increased, dumb-bells (two iron or wooden balls, connected by a handle, the whole weighing from two to five pounds each) may be employed, and the same exercises as before may be gone through with them.

12. How often each single movement should be repeated is indicated by the three numbers accompanying each figure. The first number shows the number of repetitions at first; the second that after two or three weeks; and the third that after six or eight weeks' practice. The last number is to be regarded as the limit during the rest of the practice. Each individual case, however, may require in alteration in the number of repetitions, and the middle number will be to many the normal limit, which they must not exceed; particularly as the three numbers given are based on the calculation of the normal muscular strength of a man in his best years. For people above sixty, for those weak in muscle, or very obese, for the female sex, and for children, about one half, or at the most two thirds of the amount will be sufficient. Those also, who perform the exercises for local

affections only, should not exceed the limit just given. It stands to reason that old age requires the exercise of every part of the body, so far as may be practicable. It is a great mistake, therefore, for elderly people to suppose that the greatest possible amount of rest will keep them in health. Although such persons cannot bear the same degree of fatigue as the young, a suitable amount of regular and varied exercise is necessary, if health is to be preserved and life prolonged.

13. Let me here emphasize once more the value and efficacy of (a) hydropathy; (b) a system of non-stimulating diet, at least in most cases; and (c) massage; and the desirability of adopting those systems in addition to curative gymnastics. A person, who has no knowledge of curative gymnastics, and their effect, had better leave them alone, in case of severe illness; as he will perhaps only do himself harm by attempting them. . . .

14. How many times a day curative gymnastics should be practised, and how many exercises should be gone through at each practice, depends entirely on the condition of the patient. If for instance, a practice consists of only three or four exercises, (mowing movement, raising the knee, arm-thrust, sawing movement, or a few similar exercises) from one to five such practices daily will be sufficient; but if a single practice includes a greater number of exercises, the number of practices should not exceed three. The great point here is to observe what amount of exercise will best

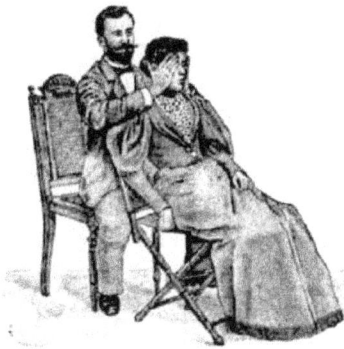

Checking a patient with an inflamed hernia for fever, and other serious symptoms, which might indicate that she requires surgery.

suit the patient's physical condition. And it must always be remembered that a beginner must be content with fewer movements than the practised gymnast can execute; and that a man in the prime of life can endure more fatigue than the young or the old.

15. When special gymnastics are employed for the cure of local complaints, it will be well to include in the practices movements which will exercise the whole of the muscles of the body, in order to bring the whole system into sympathetic and simultaneous activity. As in a set of cog-wheels, or other compound wheel-work, each single wheel performs its part when the whole is in motion, so it is with our organism; every single part of which has its office in sustaining the innermost living whole.

16. A still greater advantage is derived from curative gymnastics, when they are employed in addition to, and in connection with, massage; for the success of massage will be completed and confirmed by exercise of the muscles. That massage ought in many cases to precede curative gymnastics is demonstrated by the fact that after massage most of the movements can be performed which before it were impossible. It is not meant that every performance of gymnastics should be preceded by massage; it will be sufficient if the massage be applied once a day. It is difficult to give precise instructions in this respect; everybody must find out for himself what is adapted to his special case. It only remains to be mentioned that a proper interval of rest must be observed between the gymnastics and massage when they are combined.

17. Bed-ridden persons can execute the movements in bed, or elsewhere in a sitting or lying posture, or with the help of a second person. In the last case the movements will be passive.

18. By the use of curative gymnastics both invalids and healthy people attain, among other advantages, the blessings of refreshing sleep, improved appetite, a cheerful mind, fresh vigour of life, and increased sense of enjoyment. In practising the "arm-thrust" or hitting movements, to the front, sideways, upwards, downwards, and backwards, the fists must be kept tightly closed, and each thrust or blow should be delivered with the full and energetic extension of the arm muscles. When the muscular strength has increased, the exercises may be practised with dumb-bells, as already mentioned. They serve to supple the shoulder and elbow joints, in rheumatic affections or disabled condition of the arm muscles; they also promote healthy breathing; and should

form part of any course of general exercises. The chest-expanding movement in which energy is specially concentrated on the bringing together, and separation, respectively of the hands, is efficacious in cases of tuberculosis in the lungs, pleurodynia, asthma. It also promotes good breathing.[126]

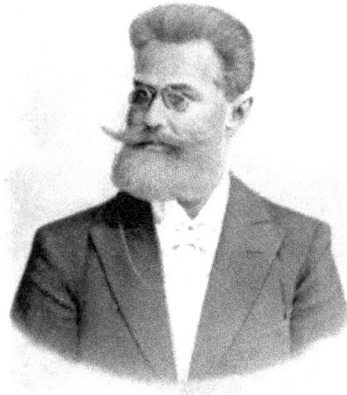

Dr. Friedrich Eduard Bilz.

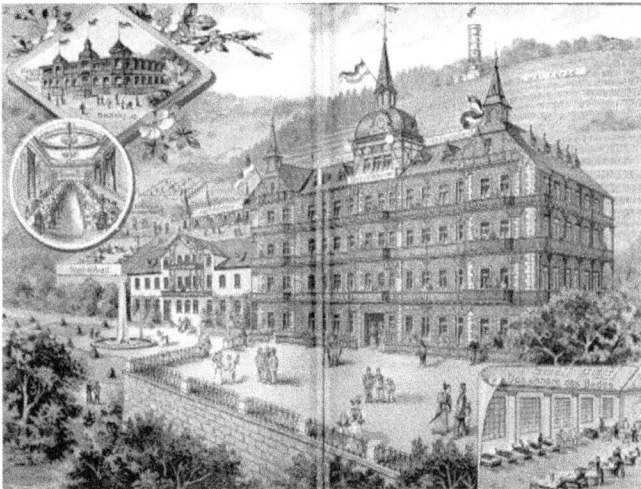

The Bilz Sanatorium, Radebeul, Dresden, Germany, 1905.

THE BILZ PROGRAM: EXERCISES FOR GENERAL HEALTH

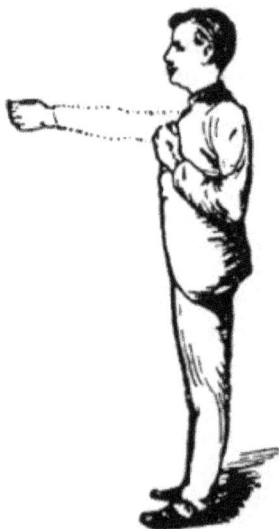

Arm thrust (hitting movement) to the front. 10, 20, 30 times.

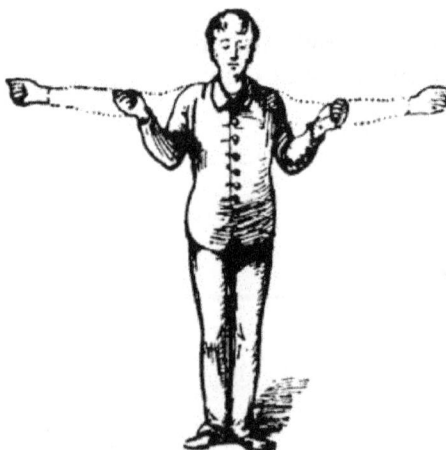

Arm thrust, sideways. 10, 20, 30 times.

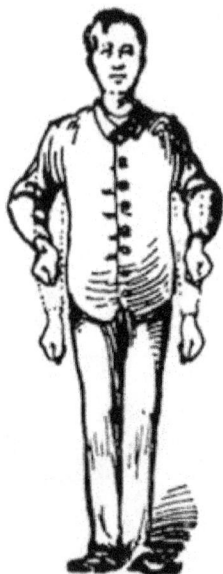

Arm thrust, downwards, 10, 20, 30 times.

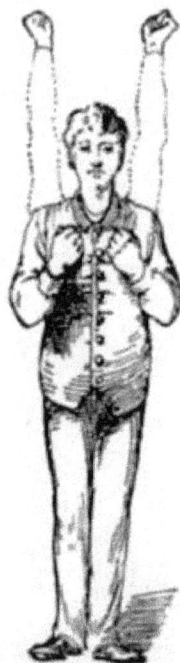

Arm thrust, upwards, 10, 20, 30 times.

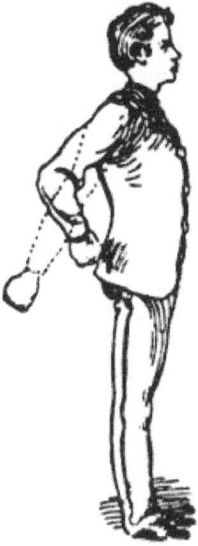

Arm thrust, to the rear,
6, 12, 18 times.

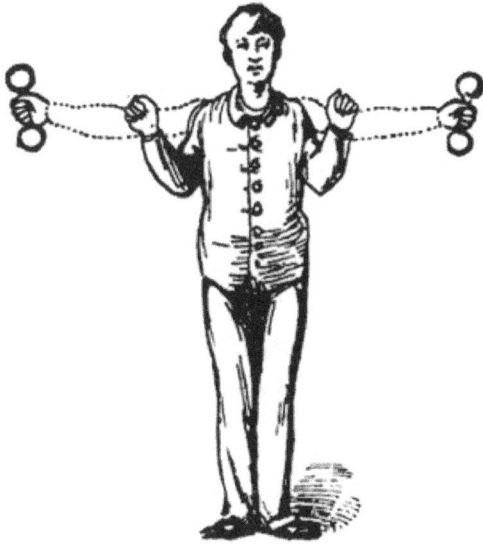

Exercise with imaginary dumbbells. 5 to 10 times.

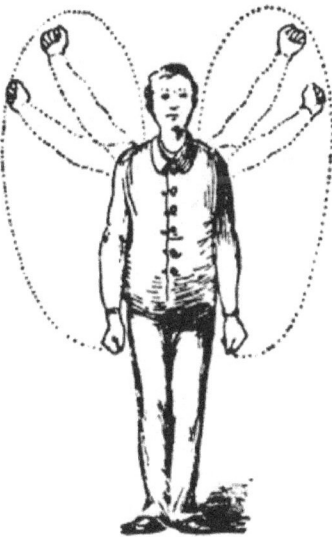

Arm circles. 8, 14, 20 times.

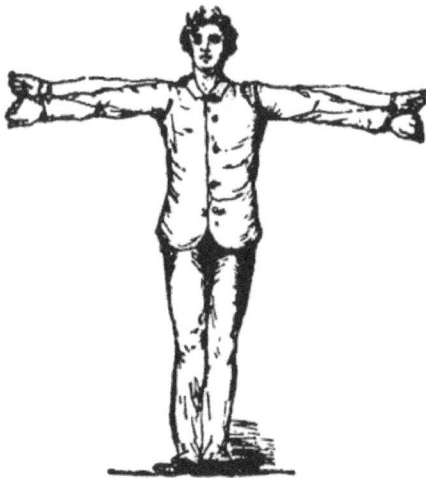

Arm rolls. 20, 30, 40 times.

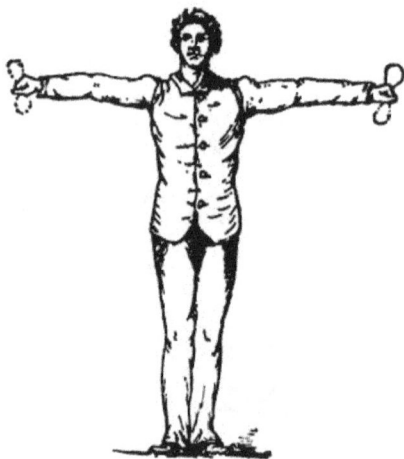

The Figure 8 Movement. 20, 30, 40 times.

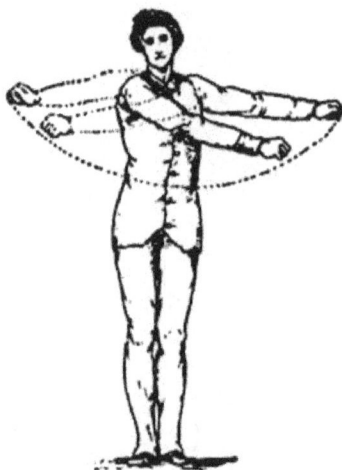

Arm Swing, sideways. 15, 25, 40 times.

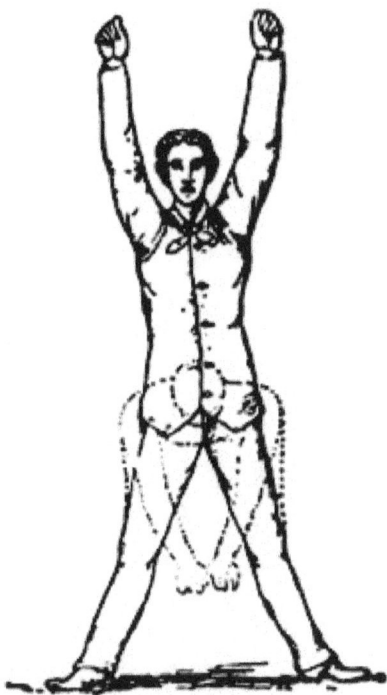

The Chopping Movement. 6, 12, 18 times.

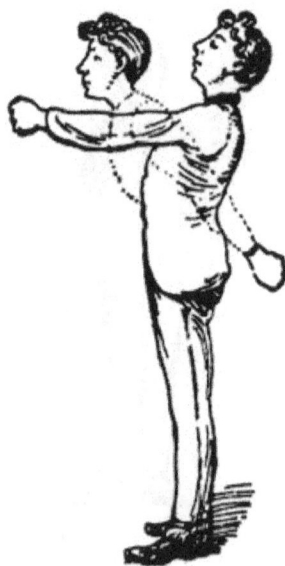

Arm Swing, to the front and rear.
15, 25, 40, times.

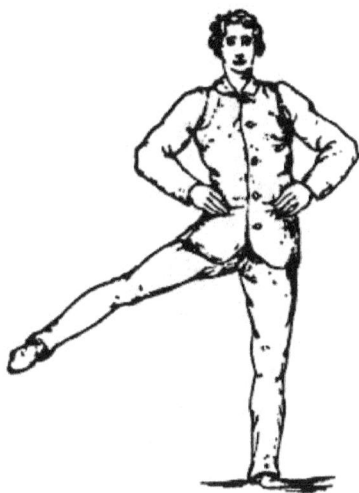

Raising the Leg Sideways. 5, 10, 18 times with each leg.

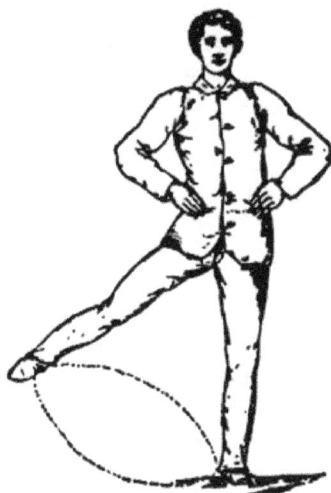

Leg Circles. 5, 8, 12 times with each leg.

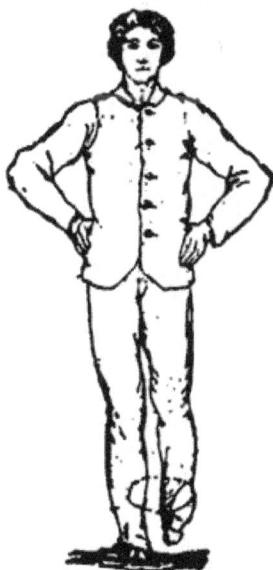

Foot Circles. 15, 25, 30 times with each foot.

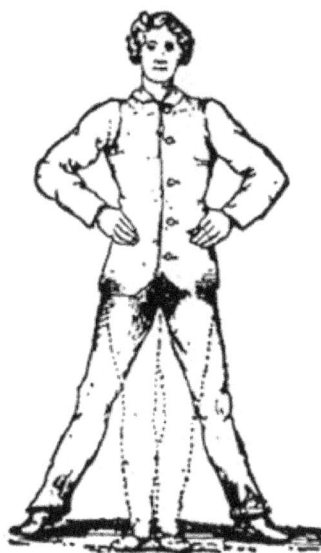

Drawing the Legs Together. 4, 6, 10 times.

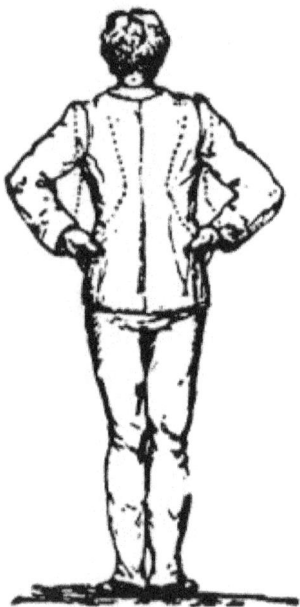

Elbows Back. 8, 12, 16 times.

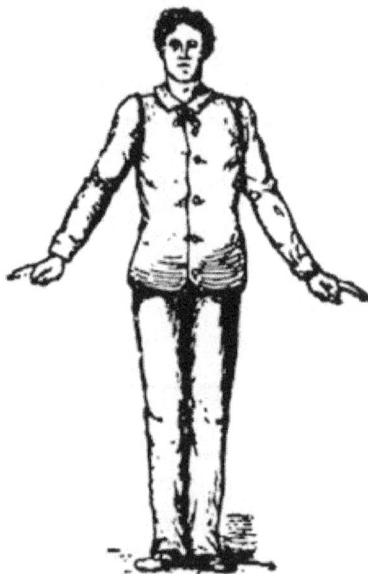

Extension and Contraction of the Fingers. 15, 20, 25 times.

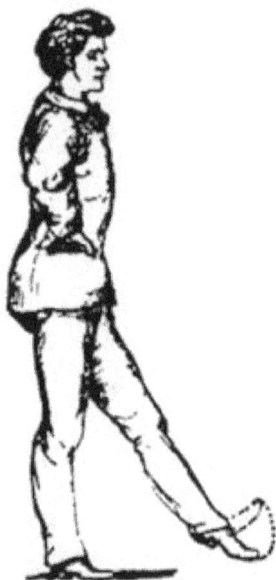

Foot Stretching and Bending. 15, 25, 35 times with each foot.

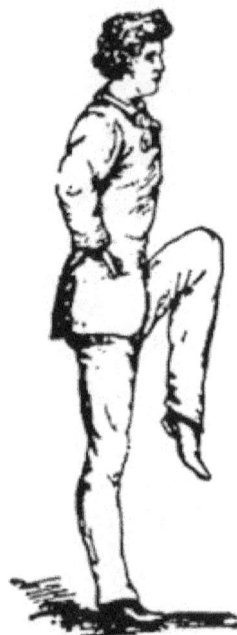

Raising the Knee. 12, 15, 18 times with each leg.

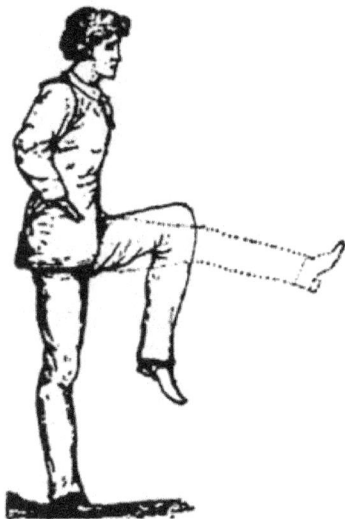

Bending and Stretching the Knee Joint to the Front. 6, 9, 12 times with each leg.

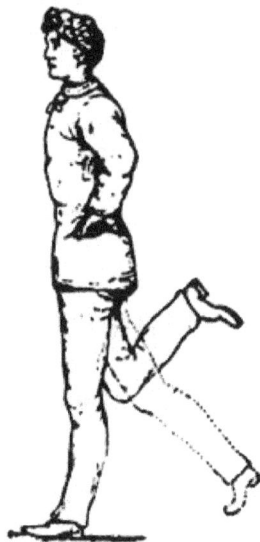

Bending and Stretching the Knee Joint to the Rear. 8, 12, 16 times with each leg.

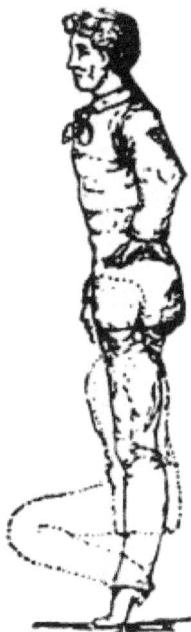

Lowering and Raising the Body. 8, 12, 20 times.

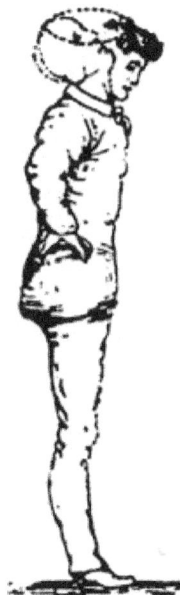

Head Circles. 8, 12, 20 times.

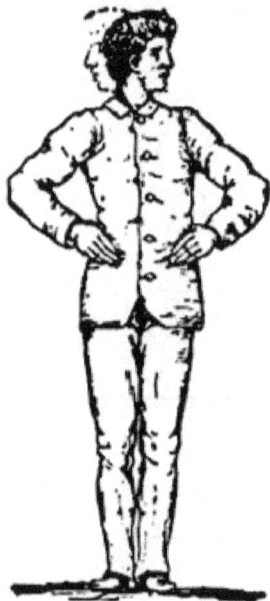

Turning the Head to Right and left. 6, 9, 12 times.

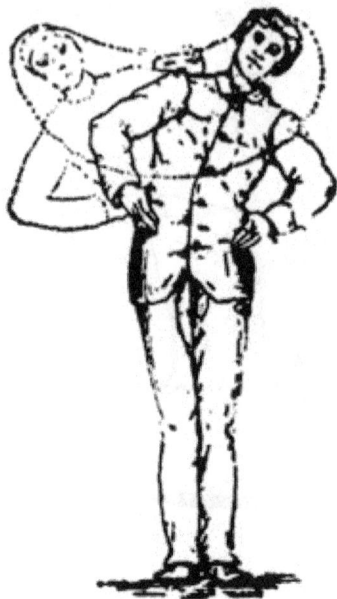

Bending the Body Sideways. 15, 25, 35 times.

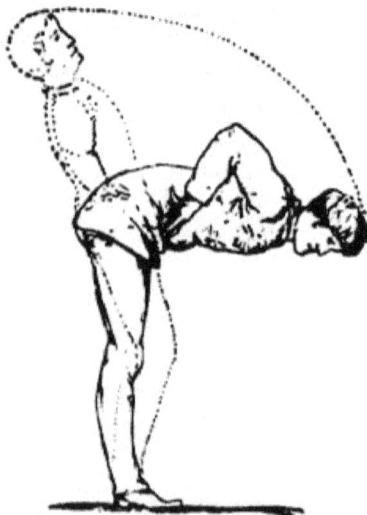

Bending the Body to the Front and Rear. 10, 20, 30 times.

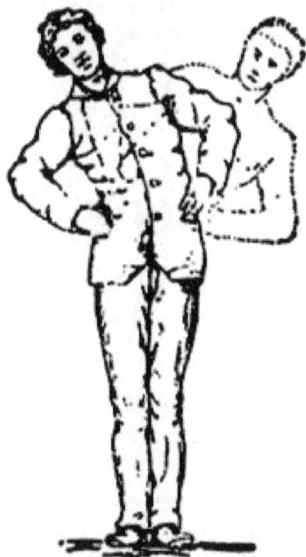

Body Circles. 6, 8, 12 times.

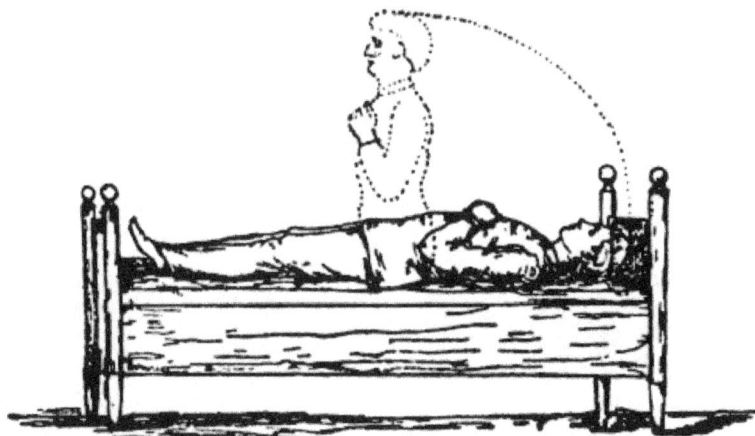

Rising From the Lying to the Sitting Position. 5, 10, 15 times.

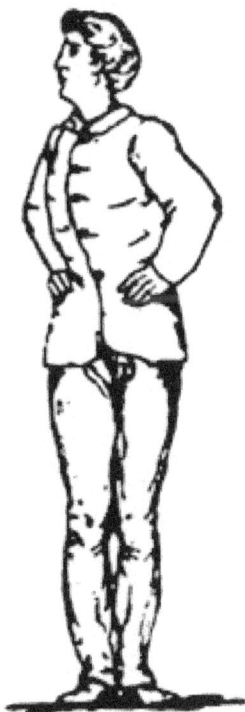

Twisting the Body. 10, 20, 30 times to and fro.

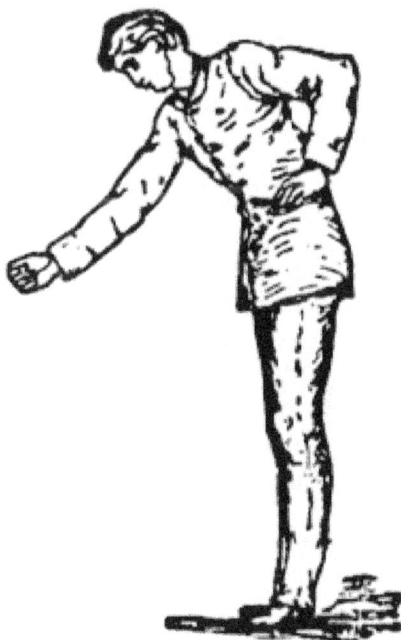

Reciprocal Sawing Movement With Both Arms at Once. 10, 20, 30 times.

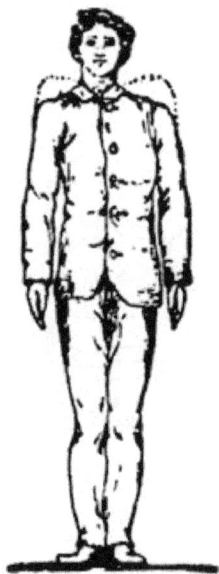

Raising the Shoulders. 20, 30, 40 times.

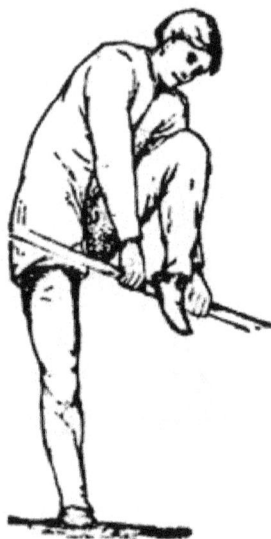

Stepping Over the Stick. 5, 8, 10 times.

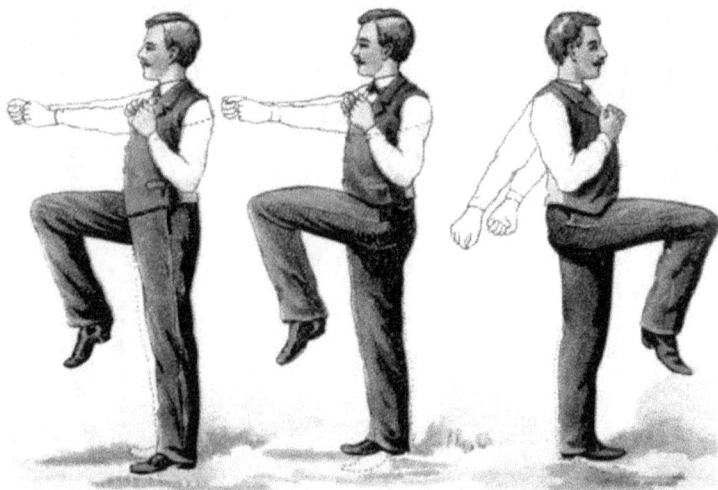

Left: Forward thrust of arms and raising right leg. Middle: Forward thrust of arms and raising left leg. Right: Backward thrust of arms and raising right leg.

WHY WEAR A TRUSS

Nearly just as popular as gymnastic exercise in the Victorian Era was the treatment of inguinal hernias with pressure, that is, with a belt or truss. In fact, it was considered mandatory. In 1889 Dr. Marcy writes:

☛ **If cure is to be effected by a truss, it must bring, and continue to hold the sides of the mouth of the sac together, so as to prevent its being opened by the insinuation of the viscera, and in time cause adhesion, and obliteration of the sac.**[127]

Dr. George Hayward writes in his 1852 book *Permanent Cure of Reducible Hernia*:

☛ **George O. Pond, M.D., of Griggsville, is confident that he has effected a cure, by means of pressure, in a number of cases of inguinal hernia. Stagner's truss is the instrument by which the pressure has been applied; and of twenty cases he thinks that seven-eighths have been permanently cured. That pressure is one of the most important modes of treating hernia, with a view to a radical cure, there is no doubt. . . . Though there is nothing new in this communication, it is nevertheless valuable, as it affords additional evidence of the power of one of the means employed to remove this infirmity.**[128]

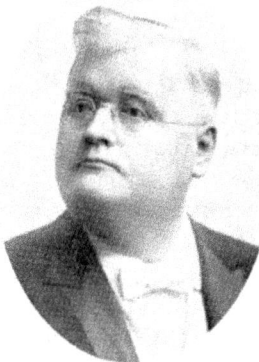

Dr. Henry Lindlahr.

Most Victorian doctors, however, used a combination of the truss and exercise, as well as an assortment of other proven remedies, including such practices as herbs,[129] acupuncture,[130] massage,[131] hydrotherapy,[132] mud baths, and Epsom salts.[133] In his 1919 book *Practice of Natural Therapeutics*, Dr. Henry Lindlahr makes the following remarks about treating inguinal hernia naturally:

☛ **These ruptures should be protected with a well-fitting truss. This has to be removed daily for cleansing of the parts. Appropriate exercises, passive and active,** together with cooling sitz baths and washes with cold water[134] and lemon juice are the best remedies for these, as well as of other forms of rupture.[135]

THE GOUR PROGRAM: INTRODUCTION
In his 1916 book *The Therapeutics of Activity*, Dr. Andrew A. Gour writes:

☛ The victims of reducible hernia often complain of pain on exertion, of dyspepsia and often, of constipation. It is advisable to eat so as to keep the bowels open, and keep from violent exercises and sudden strains.

The only proper truss is one that does not bore into the opening from outside. All kinds of methods have been applied to hold the viscus in place, but nearly all have had an oval surface which bored into the opening and tended to enlarge it. The standard truss, with its oval or sharp surface, forces into the opening and wrestles with the mass from within which is trying to come out. The result of this wrestling match is never curative. The truss is usually made strong enough and so adjusted as to overcome the pressure of the internal mass. The result of this force either way is to keep the aperture open and permanent. No truss with a conical surface ever acted as more than an artificial support. If a cure results while the standard truss is worn it is in spite of the truss. The only correct truss or support for any inguinal hernia or traumatic rupture of the abdominal wall is a broad stout band, or a band with a flat pad attached to it that exactly fits over and closes the opening from the outside without boring in. A flat piece of wood about three-eighths of an inch thick whittled out in an oval edge, lined with silk or chamois, and attached to the band will serve properly. Such an appliance will keep the hernia from bulging, keep the parts normally within the abdomen and give the aperture a chance to close up under exercise. A proper hernial support can be made by fitting a piece of 1¼ inch rubber tape around the body, bringing it close to the pubes at the front. Then attach two narrow bands lined with chamois or silk, about one inch apart at the front, pass them between the thighs and attach them at about five inches apart at the back. With these bands so adjusted that the broad abdominal part fits snugly over the hernial area, attach the flat pad so that it will press at the internal inguinal opening. This appliance is to be worn during the day. While exercising it should be removed. (See Figure 284).

THE GOUR PROGRAM: TREATMENT

The gymnastic treatment of inguinal hernia has been used successfully by Dr. Geo. H. Taylor many years ago. The late Dr. J. W. Seaver, of Yale, contributed a very instructive article to the *Yale Medical Journal*, February, 1900, 1904, on "The Treatment of Inguinal Hernia in the Young."

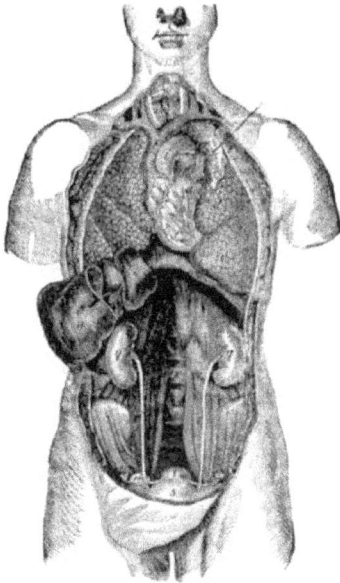

Organs of the chest and the abdomen.

In most cases it is advisable to proceed with caution, fitting the exercise to the individual, and regulating their force from gentle to strong as the patient gains. Our experience has satisfied us that the best way is to proceed progressively from gentle to strong. Dr. Seaver, whose extended experience enabled him to speak with confidence and authority, allowed even the heaviest gymnastics after the patient had practiced preliminary work for a while.

Dr. Seaver said: "It has been my experience that the patients that are most active and most anxious to take part in athletic work are the ones who repair most rapidly, while men with an aversion to physical activity do not show satisfactory results." Our experience has been such as to corroborate this statement.

The treatment of hernia is in a sense like the treatment for obesity. When the treatment is once made clear, the fact that it requires exertion on the patient's part makes it unfavorable. It is necessary to repeat the need for exercise to the patient, and to insist upon his practicing it daily. *Exercise is the only means of reinforcing the musculature of the abdomen* [my emphasis, L.S.]. **Braces, corsets, props, trusses, never have strengthened anyone.** *Besides exercise for local development of the abdominal walls, general muscular exercise is advisable* [my emphasis, L.S.]. **The home gymnastics work outlined** [below] **. . . should be taken in earnest. Any procedure tending to restore normal** [health?], **raise the viscera, develop correct carriage, etc., will relieve the pressure upon the abdominal walls and hasten permanent recovery.**

    It is sometimes advisable to allow the patient to rest a few days or weeks before commencing vigorous exercise. But during this period of rest local kneading and vibration with the proper application of cold water will always prove beneficial.

    In the application of exercises, those are best which particularly tax the oblique fibers of the abdominal muscles. [See Chapter Four for detailed information on this topic, L.S.]

THE GOUR PROGRAM: EXERCISE INSTRUCTIONS

Without further details about forms and names of herniae, let us review briefly the philosophy and application of the gymnastic treatment. *It is safe to make the general statement that very seldom do herniae exist in individuals whose abdominal muscles are strong and kept in good tonic condition. We usually find that herniae exist in individuals whose general muscular systems are flabby and weak. The abdominal muscles are relaxed and offer but a weak support to the viscera. . . . In every case where special exercise is taken to cure hernia, general exercise should also be taken. The reason is obvious* [my emphasis, L.S.].

    For local effect the best types of abdominal exercises are performed with a lateral twist of the trunk, with the patient lying on the back, or the legs are drawn up from the sides, having first been placed so as to cause a contraction of the oblique fibers. *The exercises described are sufficient to cure any case of hernia that is amenable to exercise* [my emphasis, L.S.]. **They do not include the entire possible variety, but only a selection of the best and most specific. They are all chosen for their local and specific effects, keeping in mind their general effect upon the organism.**

In applying the treatment it is advisable to proceed as follows: With the patient lying on his back, feet higher than the head:

(1) Reduce the hernia.

(2) Give the necessary osteopathic procedures.

(3) The patient's knees flexed to relax the abdominal muscles, give local kneading and vibration; alternately giving kneading a few minutes, then, vibration a few seconds.

(4) Give the exercises described below. In the beginning give the first five, then, add one at each succeeding treatment until all can be practiced at one session without tiring the patient. When all have been mastered progress by increasing the number of times each movement is repeated, always stopping short of exhaustion.

(5) After exercising give a general manipulation of the abdomen to keep the bowels active. Stimulate the liver by rhythmic pressure, percussion and vibration.

(6) Make sudden applications of cold water or ice bag over the inguinal region to cause contraction before putting on the supporting elastic pad.

As soon as possible urge the patient to lay aside the supporting pad. In a short time the abdominal muscles will be toned up to a degree that will render artificial support unnecessary for hours at a stretch. These periods will increase in length as the tonicity of the muscles is restored. When the patient feels capable he should go without the support, though he should carry it with him to put on in case of need. In a few months, even this precaution will be unnecessary [my emphasis, L.S.].

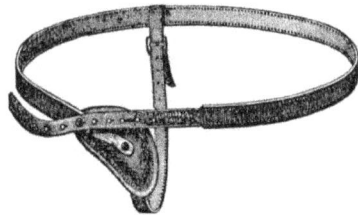

Victorian German truss, with perineal band.

While exercising to cure hernia the patient should lie on his back on an inclined table, the feet higher than the head. An incline of 10 or 15 degrees is about right. In this position gravity prevents the intestines from bulging out during the exercises.

[Important note: If you have back problems, particularly lower back issues or pain, consult your doctor before attempting Dr. Gour's exercises. Many of them are quite vigorous and could exacerbate any spinal problems you already have. L.S.]

Healthy Food Plants

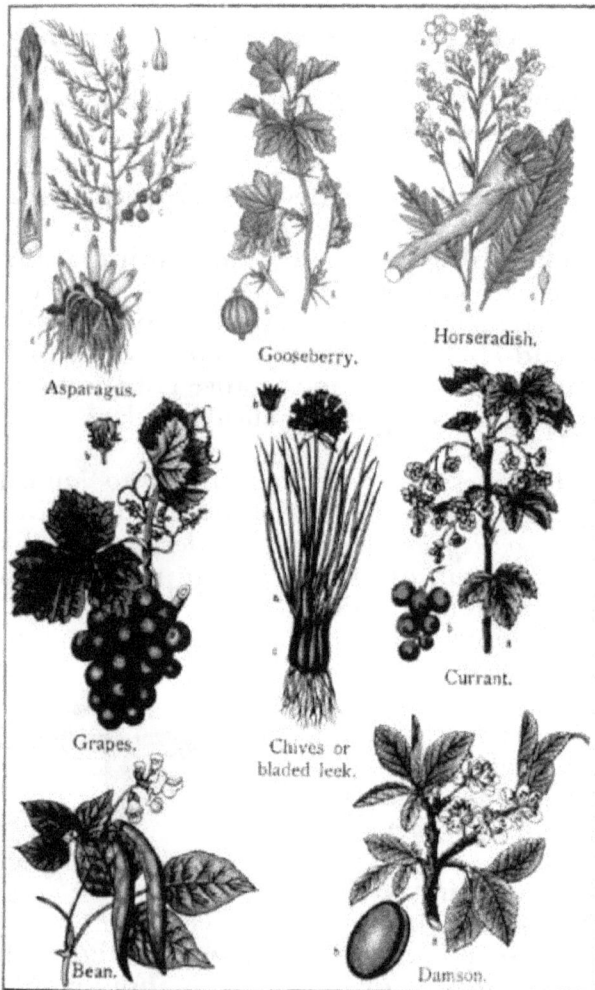

More edible vegetation used by Victorians to improve fitness and help heal inguinal hernia.

THE GOUR PROGRAM: THE EXERCISES

1. Patient lying on the back, the legs apart, the arms extended back along the head and the hands grasping the sides of the table. The operator resists as the patient draws the knee of the afflicted side up to his chest. (Illus. 285.) This is repeated a number of times. For the sake of general effect upon the abdominal muscles it is well to flex both knees, with or without resistance.

2. Patient lying on his back, knees bent and apart. The operator offers resistance as the patient brings them together. (Illus. 286.)

3. Patient lying on his back, hands grasping the sides of the table back of his head, he flexes the knees up to his chest and straightens the legs to the left, then, he flexes them again and straightens them to the right, and so on a number of times. This exercise needs no assistance or resistance and particularly affects the oblique muscles of the abdomen.

4. Patient lying on his back, legs far apart, hands grasping the table back of the head. As he elevates the legs he draws the feet together so that they touch at vertical position. As he lowers the legs he gradually spreads them apart again.

5. Reverse leg swimming. The patient is lying on the back, hands grasping the sides of the table beyond the head. He spreads the legs apart, bends the knees up to the chest as he brings the legs together and then straightens the legs out, while they are close together; and repeats the entire motion a few times, the feet are kept off the table throughout the movement. (Illus. 287.)

6. Circle the knees, keeping the feet off the table. The patient is lying as for above exercises. He flexes the knees up to the chest, carries them out to the side and then downward as he straightens them out, then, continuing in one movement he carries the legs around to the right and gradually flexes the knees as he completes the circle. This is repeated a few times without interruption, then, in reverse order the knees are carried to the right, downward, to the left and up to flexion, and so on. When this circling is done as in the first case, it effects chiefly a right inguinal hernia, and in the second case, a left inguinal, although the movement benefits and strengthens the entire abdominal walls.

7. Lying as for above movements, feet together, the patient elevates the legs and spreads them apart as they go up, bringing them together as they are lowered again.

8. Patient lying as for above movement, he raises the legs to vertical and, keeping them close together, knees straight and feet pointed, lowers them out to the left (Illus. 288), then elevates them to vertical and lowers them to the right, and so on. This is a valuable exercise to strengthen the abdominal walls, elevate the viscera, and reduce the size of the waist. To effect the hernia side especially, the legs are lowered and elevated from the afflicted side most. For instance, supposing there is a left inguinal hernia, the legs may be lowered twice or three times to the left, to once to the right.

9. Patient lying and grasping sides of table as for above exercises, he raises the legs to vertical, keeping the knees straight, toes pointed, and carries them down and outward to the left, then straight down without touching the table, over to the right and upward to vertical again, describing as large a circle as possible with the feet. This circling is done going down to the right, from vertical position, or in reverse order. It should be repeated several times in either direction in a continuous movement without resting the feet. To effect the hernia side particularly, perform the last half of the circle, that is, the lifting of the legs, to that side, and repeat twice or three times in that direction to once in the opposite.

10. Patient lying, with the hands on the hips, the feet strapped or held down, keeping the head back, he flexes up to sitting position. (Illus. 289.) This movement, as well as the two following may be made more difficult by placing the hands at the shoulders, or locking the fingers behind the head, keeping the head in line with the trunk and the elbows well back as the body is flexed upward.

11. The feet held down as for Exercise 10, hands on the hips; to affect a right inguinal hernia, the patient turns the shoulders as far as possible to the left, so as to twist the trunk and place the strain particularly at the right inguinal region. The trunk is kept twisted as it is flexed up a few times. (Illus. 290.) To affect a left inguinal hernia the trunk is twisted to the right and kept so during the exercise.

12. The feet held down as for the above two exercises,

the hands on the hips. The patient flexes the trunk half way up and, holding it there, the head in line with the body, the shoulders well back, he twists to the left and forward, or to the right and forward, a few times. The turning is done opposite to the hernia side. This exercise should be done to both sides, to strengthen the entire abdominal region, but, it is best to especially effect the hernia side by turning twice or three times to the opposite, to once on the same side as the hernia.[136]

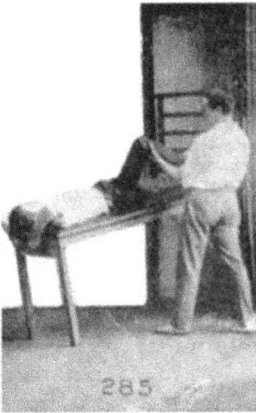

Illustration 285.

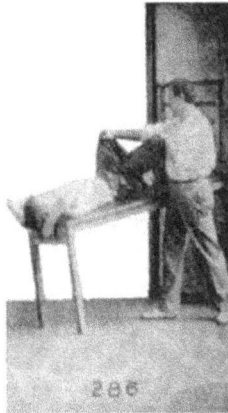

Illustration 286.

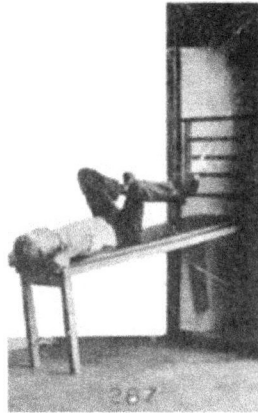

Illustration 287.

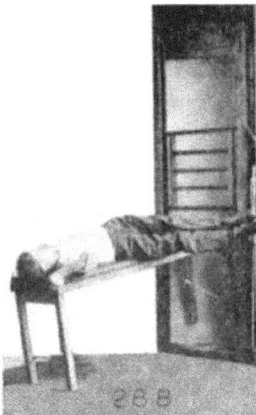

Illustration 288.

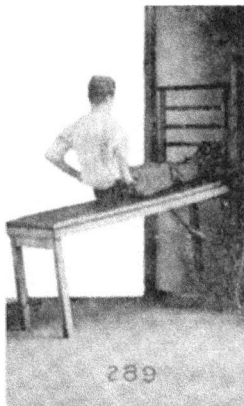

Illustration 289.

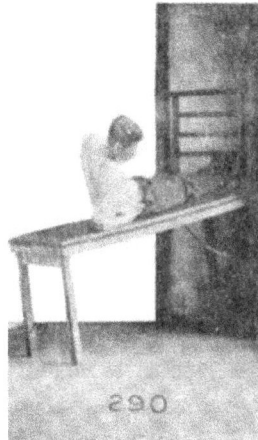

Illustration 290.

OAK BARK HERNIA HEALING METHOD

Juxtaposed against the Victorian gymnastics cure, I came across the following natural herbal cure from the year 1832. The author, James Johnson, writes that after perusing the confusing literature surrounding hernias:

☛ . . . we gladly turn to a prospect more cheering—that of *curing herniæ (reducible) in men, women, and children, without any surgical operation at all* [my emphasis, L.S.]. It is well known that the skin and other textures of an animal, when dead, are hardened and strengthened by tanning—why not tan them alive ? The idea has been long acted on, as far as the stomach is concerned. That organ we are daily in the habit of tanning with bark, steel, astringent wines, etc. The transition was very natural to the parts through which a hernia descends.

For many years past our author has used for reducible herniæ "a strong decoction of oak bark with wonderful success." Now, although we do not deny that the success might be wonderful, yet we do not like the expression, "wonderful success," from the mouth of a regular surgeon. Be that as it may, we think the proposal, as it is perfectly harmless, is well worthy of a trial, and we freely contribute to make the measure extensively known.

A few pounds of oak bark are to be macerated in a sufficient quantity of cold water, for twelve or twenty-four hours, and then the bark and solution must be put into a larger vessel, and kept at the boiling temperature over a gentle fire for two or three days, adding, when required, boiling water, from time to time, so that the bark may be always covered. The solution should be ultimately strained, and evaporated to the consistence nearly of an inspissated [thickened] juice. When used it should be warmed, to suspend the astringent matter. The hernia being previously reduced, the groin is to be bathed with the decoction, and the truss applied, three or four times a day. *Mr. Lizars has cured hernia of many years standing, in this way, in the course of a few weeks* [my emphasis, L.S.]. In general, however, it requires a perseverance of three months. This invaluable remedy was first mentioned to our author by a merchant, who cured himself after having laboured under the disease for many years.[137]

Medicinal Herbs

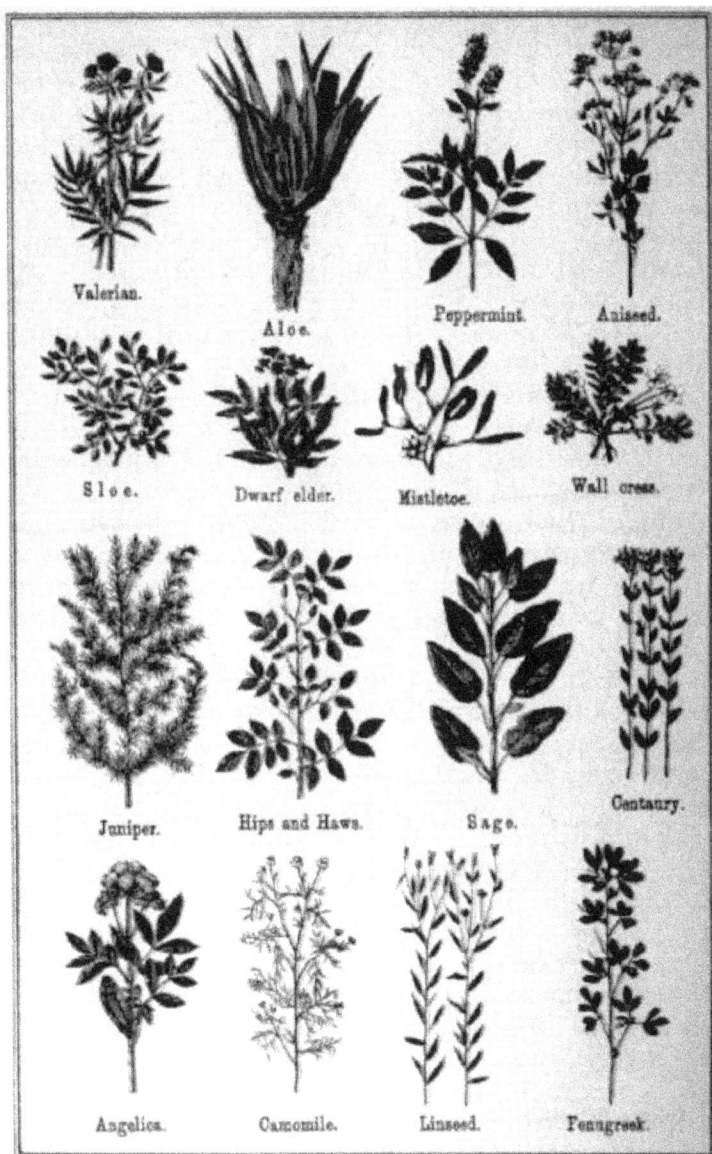

Medicinal herbs used by Victorians to improve fitness and help heal inguinal hernia.

HOMEOPATHIC HERNIA HEALING METHOD

In his 1878 book *Homeopathic Therapeutics*, Victorian naturopath Dr. Samuel Lilienthal prescribed the following remedies for various kind of hernias, including inguinal. (Warning: Please note that since many of these herbs and concoctions are not only poisonous but now also illegal, this Victorian material is presented here for historic interest only. In any case, you should consult a licensed and experienced homeopathic practitioner before attempting to use any of the potentially dangerous items below on a reducible inguinal hernia—or any other medical problem.)

☞ *Aconite*. **Violent inflammation of the parts, with burning pains in abdomen as from hot coals, extreme sensitiveness to contact; nausea, bitter bilious vomiting; anguish and cold sweat.**

Arsenicum. **Hard bloated abdomen; burning pain with anguish; sensation of coldness in upper part of abdomen; constant vomiting; great anguish, restlessness, tossing about, feeling as if the intestines became twisted; gangrene of the hernial tumor.**

Aurum. **Pressure in abdominal ring, as if hernia would protrude while sitting; protrusion of inguinal hernia, with great cramplike pains; inguinal hernia of children, umbilical hernia of children, caused by crying.**

Belladonna. **Constriction of abdomen around the navel, as if a lump or a ball would form there; feeling as if a hard body pressed from within outwards at right inguinal ring, the part not feeling hard to touch while sitting with the body bent forward; distension of abdomen, neither hard nor painful; colic, as if a spot in abdomen were seized by nails.**

Borax. **Infantile hernia; the child dreads a downward motion, is frightened by every little noise; does not thrive, brown watery diarrhea.**

Bryonia. **Hard swelling of hypochondria and around navel; painful twisting around umbilicus, with stitches, constipation.**

Calcarea carb. **Infantile hernia; considerable distension of abdomen, with colic; constant gurgling in abdomen; very open fontanelles, perspires freely about head when sleeping.**

Carbo veg. **Great anxiety, with uneasiness in abdomen; meteorism, with loud rumbling, fetid or odorless flatus;**

clothing oppresses, can hardly be endured; abdomen feels as if banging heavily; walks bent.

Cocculus. Lacerating sensation in intestines; distension of abdomen; vomiting, with bruised pain in intestines, great weakness, and inability to stand.

Colocynthis. Pain in groin, like from hernia, and on pressure sensation as if hernia would recede; abdomen distended and painful.

Lachesis. When gangrene threatens in strangulated hernia, the skin covering the hernial tumor is mottled or dark; pain across the abdomen; contractive sensation in abdomen; cutting, lacerating, burning pains in abdomen; hernia exceedingly sensitive, will not admit handling.

Lycopodium. Hernia, right side; full distended abdomen, with cold feet; grumbling and gurgling in abdomen; spasmodic contraction in abdomen; lacerating stitches in hernia.

Nitric acid. Inguinal hernia, also of children; drawing pain in abdomen, with shuddering; frequent pinching and rumbling in abdomen, which is excessively sensitive.

Nux moschata. Umbilical hernia; abdomen enormously distended; cutting pinching about navel, better from pressure; sore navel, even ulcerated.

Nux vom. Strangulated hernia; bruised pain in bowels, as if they were raw and sore; frequent protrusion of inguinal hernia, with red or yellowish foci; some tenderness from pressure on the tumor; nausea, vomiting, constipation.

Opium. Redness of face, distension of abdomen, vomiting of putrid matter, or of fæces and urine; pain in abdomen, as if intestines were cut to pieces.

Plumbum met. Incarcerated hernia; intussusception, with colic and fecal vomiting; inflammation and gangrene of the bowels; violent colic, abdomen drawn in, as if by a string, to the spine; excessive pain in abdomen, especially round the umbilicus.

Psorinum. Inguinal hernia; pain through right groin when walking; abdomen distended.

Silicea. Inguinal hernia; the child is very tender to the touch around the tumor.

Sulph. acid. Colic, with sensation as if a hernia would protrude; violent protrusion of an inguinal hernia; sour vomit, first water, then food; vomiting of drunkards.

Veratrum album. **Incarcerated hernia, not inflamed, antiperistaltic action, hiccough, cold sweat, nausea, with sensation of fainting and violent thirst; intussusception of bowels, great anguish, rushes about bent double, pressing the abdomen; cold feeling in abdomen, great sinking of strength, and empty feeling.**[138]

Thus ends our review of Victorian inguinal hernia treatments. In the next chapter I combine the knowledge, information, and experience of the aforementioned Victorian hernia doctors with my own in the formulation of a modernized self-treatment program; one that will be more readily understandable to individuals living in our hectic, fast-paced, electronic age.

Medicinal Herbs

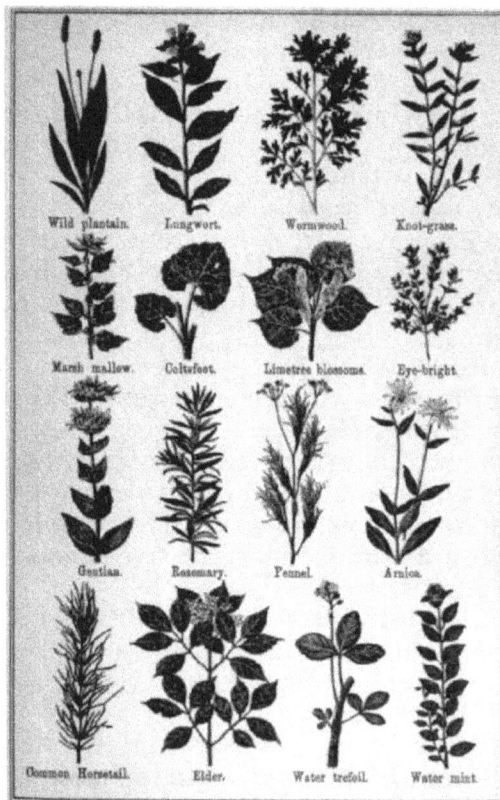

Medicinal herbs used by Victorians to improve fitness.

4

SEABROOK'S MODERN HERNIA SELF-TREATMENT PROGRAM

THE SEABROOK PROGRAM: INTRODUCTION

The foregoing chapters have given us a fascinating and educational look at the anatomy, causes, and nonsurgical healing of inguinal hernia, as described and prescribed by both mainstream and naturopathic-oriented Victorian doctors. While there is much to glean from this material for both the medical professional and the layperson, the nature of Victorian writing, with its long paragraphs, archaic words, and detailed flowery language, can be taxing for modern people, and thus difficult to follow.

To this end, I have taken this great wealth of Victorian information and both distilled it and combined it with my own knowledge and personal experience, to create a more streamlined 21st-Century plan to treat inguinal hernia without pills or scalpels. This chapter is wholly devoted to this updated, modernized natural healing program. In doing so, I am merely following the teaching of famed philosopher and advocate of the scientific method, Francis Bacon,

☛ **who in the name of true science, demanded that no inquiry that promised utility to mankind, should remain unsubjected to experiment . . .**[139]

RECAP OF REQUIREMENTS

Before we begin, let us recap the all important qualifications that must be met by those embarking on the self-healing journey. It is assumed that:

❶ You have an inguinal hernia.

❷ Your inguinal hernia is reducible; that is, you can manually push it back into your abdomen. (As repeatedly noted, irreducible hernias are, as are all other types, outside the scope of this book.)

❸ You want to avoid surgery due to pain, cost, recovery time, etc.

❹ You are an adult; that is, 18 or older. (Hernias in children, as well as non-inguinal, irreducible hernias in adults, *always* require the attention of a medical specialist. As mentioned earlier, Dr. Gour states very clearly that **"unless the sac can be reduced with the contents out of the inguinal canal into the abdominal cavity, the case is surgical and requires radical treatment."**[140]

❺ You have been examined by a qualified health provider who has determined that you are fit for a self-healing hernia treatment.

❻ You are a patient, self-regulated, self-motivated, disciplined person who is willing to make the necessary lifestyle changes and allow the required time for healing to take place.

❼ You have read the disclaimer at the front of this book.

MY APPROACH TO HEALING

My approach to healing, not just reducible inguinal hernia, but all manner of ailments, can be summarized as follows:

1. Your health is your responsibility, and your ill-health is your responsibility; not your doctor's or anyone else's. No one will ever care about your body, mind, or health as much as you do. Thus it is your obligation to learn as much about your body and healthy living as you can. If you want perfect health, no one can achieve this for you except you yourself. You create your own ease and you create your own dis-ease. It really is that elementary. While others can assist you in many positive and wonderful ways, ultimately, wholly relying on others in this regard will only postpone your good. In order to heal, it is you who must do the "heavy lifting."

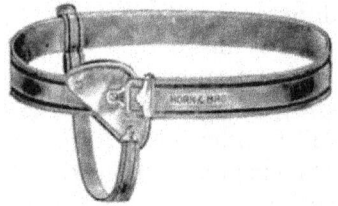

Victorian elastic truss with German pad.

2. Doctors do not heal you. Drugs and medications do not heal you. Surgery does not heal you. Your immune system is what heals you, and your immune system is controlled by your subconscious mind, which in turn is governed by God (or Nature, if you will). Understanding this is all-important because your subconscious mind operates according to your most deeply held and most consistent beliefs, feelings, and thoughts. It then physically manifests or produces them as your environment, experiences, and conditions. These, of course, include your health. When you come to completely understand these connections, it will transform your life *and* greatly aid you in healing your hernia.[141]

3. The body's natural state is health.[142] Ill-health is an imbalance of that state. If given the proper tools and time, our immune system wants to—and will automatically—restore our body's equilibrium. This is not a "miracle." It is pure science, the proof for which can be seen when you cut your finger: if you clean the wound and care for it, the cut will begin to seal up almost immediately. The same auto-healing process occurs inside you body as well, though, because it is hidden it is not as noticeable. While in some cases drugs and surgery can help, as mentioned, they do not actually heal anything. More generally medications merely provide a placebo effect while suppressing symptoms. As for cutting into the flesh, this method simply removes diseased tissue. Both of these approaches can give our immune system time to re-balance our health. But because of their negative and often toxic, even lethal, side effects, in many cases drugs and surgery actually interfere with this natural healing process. The more you know about your health, and how the mind and body work together, the more confident you will be when it comes time to decide which direction to take in healing your inguinal hernia: medical or natural, or a combination of both. Choose wisely.

INSTRUCTIONS
Let us now plunge into what I believe are the vital physical, mental, and spiritual ingredients of inguinal hernia healing.

WEIGHT
If you are overweight this could be the actual cause of your inguinal hernia, as numerous Victorian doctors in this very book assert. Even if it is not (and, as we have seen, it is usually impossible to determine the exciting cause), being overweight will hamper any progress you hope to make toward treating your hernia, for the extra weight around your middle will help pull down and stretch

out your already weakened abdominal musculature. As we have seen, the major factor in eliminating an inguinal hernia is to tighten not loosen these muscles.

Obesity also creates a build up of fatty tissue in your abdominal cavities, which in turn affects the delicately balanced tension inside—another possible exciting cause of inguinal hernia. Thus, in 1907 Dr. De Garmo listed "fat" as one of the primary causes of this specific type of hernia:

☞ **That fat, either in excess, or suddenly acquired, is productive of inguinal hernia, is abundantly proven. It acts in several ways: (a) By increasing intra-abdominal pressure; (b) by slipping into the canal, the point of least resistance under violent muscular exertion; (c) by the formation of subperitoneal lipoma, which may descend through the canal, dragging with it a process of peritoneum which then becomes [a] hernial sac; (d) fat acquired by excessive beer drinking, has been found particularly productive of hernia, by a two-fold action. First, in the accumulation of fat; second, in causing fatty degeneration of muscular tissue. This condition makes these patients poor subjects for the curative operation, increasing the danger and diminishing the chances of permanent cure.**[143]

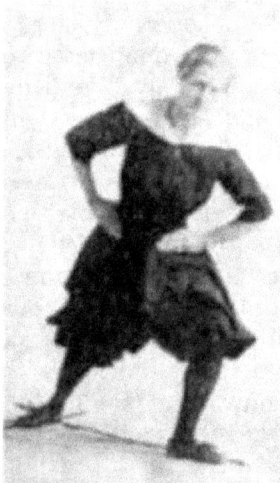

Almost any gentle exercise benefits inguinal hernia in one way or another.

In most of the books in my bibliography, excess fat is mentioned as a cause, or a contributing cause, in the formation of hernias. It was so well accepted in this regard 150 years ago that some Victorian surgical manuals recommended that surgeons try to remove "accumulations" of abnormal fat (as opposed to normal healthy fatty tissue) during hernia operations in order to help prevent reoccurrence.[144]

Decide right now to lose the necessary weight. Begin eating correctly as soon as possible. Not only will you feel and look better, but you will remove one of the greatest obstacles to healing your hernia while simultaneously increasing your overall health, quality of life, and longevity.

If you do not feel qualified to determine the proper weight for your age, height, occupation, and body type, by all means contact a doctor, dietician, or nutritionist.

POSTURE

Posture can have a profound impact on the formation of an inguinal hernia as well as preventing it from healing, which is why Dr. De Garmo lists it as one of his top nine causes of hernia.[145]

While there is endless advice concerning the correct hernia postures, it is easiest to remember this one simple rule: no slouching. When sitting, sit upright. When standing, stand upright. When walking, walk upright, leaning back ever so slightly so that the spine and pelvis tilt slightly backward.

All of this is important because in many individuals, particularly the heavyset, slouching pushes extra weight onto the anterior abdominal region, driving excess pressure into the already inherently weak tissues in that part of the abdomen. This, of course, will further complicate any healing of inguinal hernia.[146]

Sit tall. Stand tall. Walk tall.

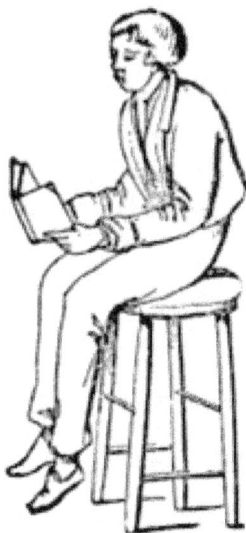

DIET

We all possess different body types and live different lifestyles. This means we each have different caloric and nutritional needs. Thus, contrary to common wisdom, there is no one diet for everyone. What works for me may not, and almost certainly will not, work for you, and vice

According to Victorian doctors, bad posture (shown here) can both exacerbate an existing inguinal hernia and cause one.

versa. Imagine someone who lives in the Arctic region of Canada trying to eat the same diet as someone who lives on the equator in Brazil, or vice versa, and you will begin to see the problem.

Having said this, I think most intelligent people can agree that whether one considers themself a carnivore, omnivore, or vegetarian, *organic natural foods* are best if one wants to maintain optimum dietary health. (The horrific toll on physical health that comes from eating chemically laced foods is well attested to throughout scientific literature. For example, foods containing artificial additives increase estrogen in men, which will inevitably lead to a host of serious health problems.)

How can you tell which foods are best for you and which are not? One easy method is to note how you feel after eating a specific food. Your body is the best judge on this score, and will inform you, usually quite quickly, as to what you should be eating and what you should not be eating. Digestive problems, headaches, edema, hives, itching, and lethargy are some of the primary indicators that you are eating the wrong foods, and that you are in fact probably allergic to several if not all of them.

What does this have to do with healing an inguinal hernia?

What you eat, how much you eat, and how often you eat all have a direct impact on hernia healing. For one thing, a constantly full or bloated lower digestive tract will strain and stretch out the tissues around your hernia, helping to prevent tightening of the muscles. For another, it is well established that good nutrition is key to building and maintaining healthy tissue. As such, some Victorian doctors attributed hernias almost solely to improper diet and poor nutrition.[147]

One of these was Dr. Lindlahr. In 1919 he discussed what he considered the main cause of hernias in newborns:

☛ **As a result of a weakly or sickly condition of the mother during pregnancy and of faulty prenatal management, many children are born ruptured** [i.e., with a hernia]. **So far I have not known a single nature cure baby** [that is, one from a mother eating a nutritious diet] **that was born ruptured. Such defects are due to weakness of the tissues. This results from mineral starvation. The tissue walls contain too much mortar (protein) and not enough building stone (mineral salts).** *Prevention of hernia, therefore, lies mainly in proper diet* [my emphasis, L.S.] **of the pregnant mother, but all the rest of the prenatal regimen described in these pages is of great importance in preventing this and other ailments and deformities.**[148]

Concerning the affect of overeating and its relation to the making of hernias, Joseph H. Warren writes the following in his 1880 book *A Practical Treatise on Hernia*:

☛ **When the bowels are distended with food or air the whole front wall of the abdomen is projected forward.**

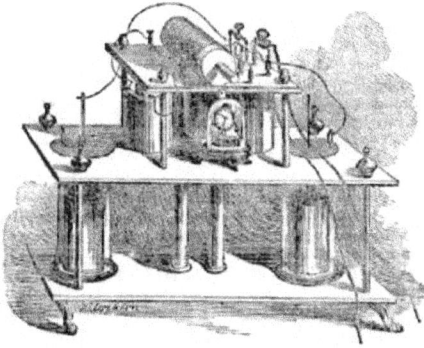

In 1864 the "Magnetic Electromotor" produced electricity that was said to be "useful in all diseases," including those related to the abdomen.

There being no vacuum and action and reaction being equal, the pressure is equally distributed over the whole of the containing parietes [parieties are the walls of a cavity; e.g., the abdominal parietes]. The mesentery is stretched to its utmost. If the sides be sound and equally resisting, the whole of the abdominal wall yields equally to the pressure and no hernia occurs; but, if one part be weak while another is resisting, that part yields to the pressure and a hernia results. The culminating point of the pressure is produced by the action of the recti and other abdominal muscles antagonizing the downward pressure of the abdomen and the inspiratory action of the lungs. The most likely, as well as the most frequent place for the abdominal walls to yield before such pressure, is in the aponeurotic structures at the side of the recti muscles, especially when the internal abdominal ring is not sufficiently strong.[149]

If you want to eliminate your hernia, it is in your best interest to build a new menu around healthy foods. Along with this, eat small meals, cut portion sizes, do not snack between meals, do an occasional fast, do not overeat, and avoid inflammatory foods and habits. The latter category includes smoking and drinking (alcohol), as well as eating processed meats, dairy products (in particular cow's milk and cheese), food additives, fatty red meats, saturated fats (such as fried chicken, hamburgers, bologna, hot dogs), refined sugar products (sugary desserts like pastries, doughnuts, cake), and *all* processed foods (vegetable oils, margarine, bagged snacks, junk cereals, white bread, white flour pastas, cured meats, etc.). Some of these so-called "foods" can literally kill you if eaten for an extended period of time.

Nothing more need be said here, for this is not a book about food and diet. Suffice it to say that if you try your best to copy the diet of your great-grandparents, your health will improve by leaps and bounds. Better yet, consider the diet of prehistoric peoples, who ate nothing but natural organic foods throughout their entire lives. They were fortunate indeed to have lived before the invention of inorganic processing and white sugar, and before chemicals (many actually poisonous) were developed and added to foods to artificially enhance their color, texture, taste, appearance, and shelf life.[150]

In short, if you have not already, change poor eating and cooking habits to healthy ones. Eliminate foods you may be allergic to (these are usually what you consider your "favorite" foods, or the ones you consume most often). Above all, avoid altered unnatural foods and replace them with unaltered natural foods. These improvements, though seemingly difficult at first, will pay huge future dividends in your general health and sense of well-being, while greatly increasing your chances of healing your hernia.

THE HERNIA BELT

Your inguinal hernia cannot and will not heal if it continually pops out of your abdominal wall. Even if it protrudes only once a day, this will slow and even prevent total healing. For, as Dufour writes,

☛ **if [a] cure be attempted it can be effected only by restoring the containing parts to their original strength and adequateness.**[151]

This means investing in a quality, well made hernia belt, or truss as Victorians called it, one that *completely* prevents your hernia from poking through its muscular enclosure. Your truss must fit snugly but remain both comfortable and wearable for long periods *while holding your hernia in place at all times*. This means it must retain the hernia during activities such as walking, sitting, lying down, walking upstairs, bending backward and forward, coition, coughing, etc.[152] Of this topic, Dr. Hayward writes in 1852:

☛ **In the treatment of** [reducible inguinal] **hernia in this way** [that is, wearing a hernia belt that exerts the correct pressure on the inguinal area], **it is of the utmost importance that protrusion should not be allowed to take place at any time; "for if the hernia once descends during the wearing of the truss," as Sir Astley Cooper well remarks, "the cure must be considered as recommencing from that moment." The truss, therefore, should be worn by night as well as by day** [Note: Opinions vary as to these views, L.S.].

It is important, also, that while the pressure is sufficient to prevent the descent of any of the abdominal contents, it should not be enough to cause any considerable degree of inflammation. This would not only require the truss to be laid aside altogether, but it would also stop entirely the effusion of fibrine [a white insoluble fibrous protein]. In inguinal hernia, the pad should be so placed as to compress the inguinal canal; and at the same time great care should be taken to avoid pressing the spermatic cord against the pubis.

A radical cure will not be effected in this way, unless the compression is continued for a length of time. . . . [M]ore benefit is derived from compression in such cases than from anything else, and persons in this situation are not safe without it.[153]

Furthermore, according to a prestigious Victorian medical committee:

☛ . . . compression [that is, wearing a hernia belt], **when properly employed, is, in the present state of our knowledge, the most likely means of effecting a radical cure in the greatest number of cases.**[154]

In at least one instance Dr. De Garmo, a pro-surgery hernia physician, seems to agree, saying in 1886,

☛ **that he thought skilled mechanical appliances** [such as hernia belts] **would cure as large a percentage of herniae as any operation performed in these days.**[155]

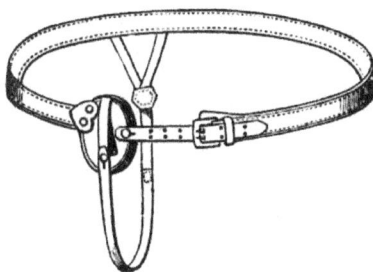

A Victorian English leather truss.

How you put on and wear your truss are two of the most important elements in hernia self-healing. In 1878 Dr. Agnew offered this advice:

☛ **Before applying the instrument** [truss] **the person should assume the supine posture, with the shoulders elevated and the limbs drawn up** [i.e., knees bent], **so as to** relax the parts and to allow the contents of the sac to be pressed back into the abdomen. The hips should then be raised and the truss carried around the pelvis in the position which will be shown under the special forms of hernia. The strap being made fast, the patient may rise from the bed and assume the standing position. To be certain that the hernial passages are thoroughly secured, the patient may cough, bend forwards and backwards, stoop down with the limbs widely separated, and finally sit down with the limbs crossed. If these different tests be applied without the hernia escaping beneath the truss, the instrument may be accepted as a proper one.[156]

HERNIA BELT BRAND

I do not recommend hernia belt brands. Not only because there are countless types and makes to choose from, but more specifically because everyone's body is different, and fit and comfort are key to proper healing. As Dr. De Garmo writes in 1886:

☛ One kind of truss cannot be adapted to all cases, and great skill and experience are necessary in the selection for each individual patient.[157]

If you are like many hernia sufferers, you will probably end up trying a number of different labels and styles before you discover one that is right for you. Once you do, you may find that you require at least two hernia belts: one for exercising and showering in, and a second one for normal daily activities (working, shopping, etc.).

Assuming your hernia is reducible (this book focuses only on the hereditary disease known as reducible, congenital, inguinal hernia), you will very likely be able to remove your belt while sleeping without fear that it will pop out in the middle of the night. This will give your body a rest from the restrictive discomfort that often comes from wearing a truss for hours at a time. Experiment to see what works for you.

If you have questions about sleeping without your hernia belt, be sure to consult your doctor, for a hernia, even the seemingly benign, self-treatable, reducible inguinal type, can be (or can quickly become) a potentially problematic medical condition. Hence, it should always be taken seriously.

THE LIFESTYLE FACTOR

Stress, of one kind or another—like vitamin D deficiency—is at the root of nearly ever disease and ailment, and stress is usually a result of one's lifestyle. Thus if you want to naturally and nonsurgically treat your hernia, you must reexamine your lifestyle.

While we now know that the main cause of inguinal hernia is almost always congenital (inherited weak abdominal muscles), it is usually impossible to determine its exciting cause. When I asked my doctor what the exciting cause of mine might have been, he chuckled and said: "It could have been anything, from tying your shoes to jumping rope." In other words, no one would ever know, least of all he himself. This is, in great part, because, as we have seen, inguinal hernias begin in the womb and can take decades to form before they begin to protrude and are finally noticed.

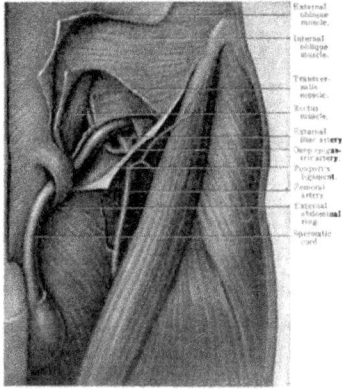

An inside look at an inguinal hernia.

Hundreds of other exciting causes are known, too numerous to mention here, but the primary ones include lack of physical fitness, poor nutrition, sneezing, yelling, fighting, lifting, bending, blowing, laughing, energetic coition, jumping, falling, straining in the bathroom, or any other kind of, what Victorian doctors called, "violent exertion." Victorian author Mark Twain got a hernia from coughing. While you will probably never discover the precise exciting cause of your own reducible inguinal hernia, rest assured that it almost certainly manifested due to some form of stress.

Knowing this, it behooves the hernia sufferer to do all he or she can to create a peaceful wholesome lifestyle, one that is gentle on both the mind and on the body; one that is conducive to both mental and physical health. Old negative health-destroying habits should be rooted out and replaced with new positive health-giving ones. Since you are unique and your lifestyle is unique, only you (and a health professional, if need be) will know what your unwholesome habits are and how to deal with them.

There is no reason why you cannot begin to make the necessary adjustments this very moment. The sooner you do, the sooner you will find your inguinal hernia improving, and hopefully shrinking and eventually disappearing—the goal of this book.

THE MIND & HEALING

Wired to our autonomic nervous system and other involuntary bodily systems, our subconscious mind regulates our immune system, which is in turn responsible for healing. While much of the subconscious mind operates on "auto-pilot" (involuntarily regulating physical functions like our heartbeat, breathing, and digestion), science proved centuries ago that the subconscious mind is also highly amenable to suggestion—as the mental state known as hypnosis clearly shows.[158]

Suggestions can come from an external source, for example, a TV show, a billboard, a book, or the words of a preacher, politician, or hypnotist. More importantly for our purposes, suggestions can originate internally; that is, in the form of *auto-suggestion*: using our own thoughts, words, and beliefs to influence our physical conditions.

In his 1916 book *The Law of Psychic Phenomena*, Victorian mental science researcher Thomas Jay Hudson states unconditionally that:

☛ **Properly understood and applied, auto-suggestion supplies a means of enabling every one to heal himself . . . Many of the pain and ills to which the average man is subject can be cured by this means.**[159]

Auto-suggestions are most commonly planted in the subconscious mind by way of affirmations: a positive statement or thought made by the conscious mind, such as "I am healed," "I am improving everyday," "I feel fantastic." The subconscious mind, which never sleeps, tires, or fails, is constantly listening to what we are thinking consciously; likewise it absorbs our most deeply held beliefs and our most consistent thoughts. It then takes these beliefs and thoughts and uses them to create our environment, our experiences, and our circumstances.

The astute reader will immediately recognize the importance of this knowledge: Whatever thoughts our conscious mind programs our subconscious mind with will eventually become what we perceive as our physical reality, including physical health; for **"the brain can influence even the organic functions."**[160] Hence, Saint Paul makes the following recommendation:

☛ **. . . whatsoever things are true, whatsoever things are honest, whatsoever things are just, whatsoever things are pure, whatsoever things are lovely, whatsoever things are of good report; if there be any virtue, and if there be any**

praise, think on these things.[161]

The more enlightened doctors of the Victorian age likewise taught their patients the importance of positive thinking. One of these was Dr. Henry Lindlahr, who promoted natural healing methods that combined fresh air, fasting, water treatment, homeopathic medicines and herbs, massage, and mental attitude, the latter for which he gave the following advice:

☛ **Courage, serenity, and presence of mind** [are] **important factors** [in healing]. **Fear and anxiety intensify disease conditions, poison the secretions of the body and inhibit the action of the healing forces. . . . The right mental and emotional attitude of relatives and friends** [also] **exerts a powerful influence upon the patient.**[162]

LAW OF ATTRACTION

Humans have been aware of, not only how our thoughts dramatically affect our health, but more importantly the amazing "mind over matter" powers of our subconscious mind, since prehistoric times. Variously called the Law of Reciprocity and the Law of Attraction, it was known to or taught by, among thousands of others, Jesus,[163] Buddha, Krishna, Moses, Zoroaster, Plato, Lao Tzu, Pythagoras, Saint Hildegard of Bingen, Isaac Newton, Francis

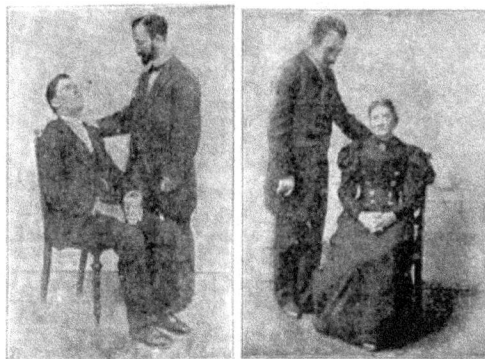

Psychotherapeutic methods like hypnosis, suggestion, and auto-suggestion have been used to heal disease for thousands of years, including inguinal hernia.

Bacon, Paramahansa Yogananda, Napoleon Hill, Johann Wolfgang von Goethe, Mahatma Gandhi, Ella Wheeler Wilcox, Winston Churchill, and Thomas Edison.[164]

The science behind using spiritual laws, like the Law of Attraction, to heal one's hernia (or any other ailment), is simple and universal: *Like attracts like*. This fundamental scientific-spiritual principle has been aptly demonstrated by scientists for many hundreds of years. One of these, the 18th-Century French physicist André-Marie Ampère, for example, discovered that:

☛ **Parallel currents in the same direction attract one another; parallel currents in opposite directions repel one another.**[165]

Because everything, including our minds and bodies, is composed of energy—which according to the First Law of Thermodynamics, cannot be created or destroyed—thoughts too are a form of energy, one that can be measured and recorded (as brain waves) on a variety of equipment, such as an electroencephalogram machine (EEG). Thus, as I write in my book *Jesus and the Law of Attraction*:

> Thoughts are things, thoughts are creators, thoughts are builders, imbued with a divine magnetism that draws everything in that is like the thoughts themselves. Operating in the invisible (spiritual) as electric waveforms, thoughts have the full capacity to manifest in the visible (physical) as material objects. For everything, from the book you are now holding, to the Universe itself, began as a thought frequency in the Divine Mind of God, becoming "the Word made flesh."[166]

AS A MAN THINKETH

Knowing the manner in which the conscious mind influences our subconscious mind gives new meaning to the biblical scripture: "As a man thinketh, so is he,"[167] for modern psychology has firmly established that you become what you think—as well as what you feel and believe.[168] *Every moment you are literally creating your own reality*. The same can be said for the science of psychotherapeutics, which, time and time again, has irrefutably demonstrated that

☛ **there is a psychic power inherent in man which can be employed for the amelioration of his own physical condition, as well as that of his fellows.**[169]

How does this power relate to hernia healing?

Because brain waves are things, thinking positive, uplifting thoughts benefits our entire mind-body complex, while thinking negative, demoralizing thoughts degrades our entire mind-body complex. This means that everyone has the mental power to heal themselves.[170]

In terms of the subject of this book, just as wrong thinking helps lead to an unhealthy life, right thinking helps lead to a healthy life, and this includes the health of your abdominal region—the site of your hernia. By consciously dwelling on, constantly affirming, and visually imagining the complete healing of your hernia, your subconscious mind responds accordingly, ultimately transforming these thoughts into reality.

You now know that the mind and body are integrally intertwined. And you now know how to use this connection to improve both your life and treat your hernia.

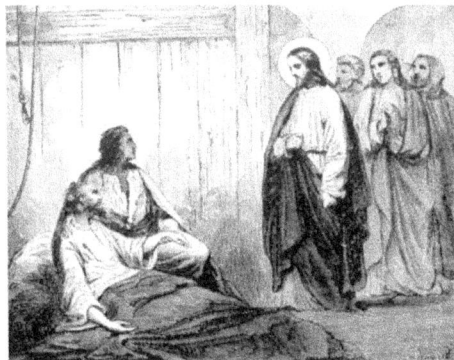

The greatest healer in history was Jesus, who, using telepathy, spiritual (i.e., mental) power, and external suggestion, cured believers of every manner of disease. This Victorian illustration depicts the Master's healing of the paralytic (Mark 2:1-12).

This power was not just granted to Jesus and other great spiritual leaders and teachers. You possess this divine ability too.[171] And you have every right to use it to heal and bless yourself—as Jesus Himself repeatedly insisted,[172] for, He enjoined: "If thou canst believe, all things are possible to him that believeth."[173] Have complete faith. Trust fully in this power.[174] And, according to both Victorian psychologists and the Master, you will be made whole.[175]

PREVENTION

If you have a pattern or history of inguinal hernias in your family line, this probably indicates a hereditary predisposition to what Victorian physicians labeled a "disease," which in this case would be inherently weak abdominal muscles and/or tissues.

If you are reading this book and do not have a hernia, or have had one and would not like to repeat the experience, you can use the instructions and exercises in this book as a prevention program. Based on my experience, and that of many others—including countless 19th-Century doctors and hernia patients—this information can and should help you avoid an occurrence or a reoccurrence.

DESCRIPTION & FOCUS

Now on to my version of the physical foundation of nonsurgical self-treatment: the Seabrook Low Impact Abdominal Exercise Program. This is something I personally developed over many months as part of my own reducible inguinal hernia treatment. It worked for me. It could work for you.

As its name implies, the program focuses on the abdomen, with special emphasis on the lower abdominal region where the inguinal ligaments and the transversus abdominus muscles (which support the abdominal wall) are located. When these tissues, as well as those surrounding them, become soft and weak (either due to heredity or inactivity, or both), it can set the stage for an inguinal hernia, or what ancient doctors inaccurately called a "rupture" in the abdominal wall. My exercises target these muscles, strengthening them and building them back up through repetitive physical movement.

While the exercises presented by Dr. Andrew A. Gour in the previous chapter were also designed to treat reducible inguinal hernia—and are thus well suited to controlling and ultimately healing this particular disease—some may find them too extreme or even violent in their effect on the body. I am speaking here of the young, the elderly, the infirm, the ill, the delicately built, and more specifically those with back (and especially lower back) problems.

My program takes a gentler approach to hernia healing, with low impact exercises that are designed to improve muscle strength while minimizing injury, pain, and distress. If you begin with my workout routine, however, eventually you may find that you are able to switch over to Dr. Gour's. And you can always go back and forth, depending on your mood and state of health.

EXERCISE INSTRUCTIONS

A) Since, like everything else in this book, you follow my exercise program at your own risk, please get approval from your doctor before embarking on it. You do not want to further impair your present hernia, or in the worst case scenario, create another hernia in a different part of your body.

B) Make sure your hernia is reduced before beginning.

C) Do your workout on an empty stomach and between meals, preferably morning (before breakfast) and late afternoon (before dinner).

D) Do your workout on a comfortable firm surface, such as a floor mat, carpet, or rug.

E) Perform the exercises calmly and slowly. No fast, jarring, or extreme actions or movements.

F) Continue to breathe normally throughout each session. Never hold your breath while exercising.

G) Do your workouts in a quiet peaceful space and in a relaxed manner whenever possible. You want to be able to completely focus on your exercises, with the fewest distractions possible.

H) Healing is not all physical. As we have seen, health begins in your mind with total belief in what you are doing, enthusiasm toward your workouts, and a clear strong view of your goals. While performing the exercises, mentally visualize your muscles building, the tissues tightening, your hernia disappearing, and your hernia belt being tossed aside.

I) The main purpose of this program is to strengthen your abdominal muscles. To aid in this process, always tighten your core muscles at the start of each exercise, then release when done. Known as "engaging the core," this vital practice is more than merely holding one's breathe, as many mistakenly believe. To truly achieve an engaged core, you must squeeze or contract all of the core muscles as if in anticipation of receiving a blow to the stomach. This activates the four key muscle sections of the abdominal area: the transverse abdominis, the internal obliques, the external obliques, and the rectus abdominis. It is these four groups which are directly or indirectly associated with inguinal hernias. Note: While engaging your core, remember to breath normally. (See F above.)

J) If you are not in shape, start off slowly. I recommend beginning with one session a day, until your body becomes accustomed to the increased exercise. Also, keep exercise repetitions (reps) to a minimum in the beginning, which will give your muscles time to adjust to the new movements. As your body builds in strength you can increase the number of both reps and daily sessions—although personally I would advise limiting your sessions to no more than two a day. See next entry.

K) Do not overdo it. Never perform any exercise to the point of exhaustion. Stop if and when you are uncomfortable, tired, or are experiencing pain or any type of soreness, irritation, or tenderness. If the discomfort does not disappear in a reasonable amount of time, contact your doctor.

L) As your muscles get stronger you may want to increase the number of reps in each exercise, as well as the duration of each exercise. Listen to your body.

M) The body responds in a remarkable manner to daily disciplined exercise, and so you will probably notice improvements within the first 24 to 48 hours. With the passage of days and weeks your abdominal muscles will strengthen, the exercises will get easier, and the program will become more enjoyable. Stick with it. Trust the process.

N) Important: Be sure to include other types of exercises in your hernia healing regimen besides those listed below and the others discussed in this book. Walking, hiking, swimming, yoga, and bicycling, for example, build overall physical and mental health while toning both the abdominal muscles and the back muscles, all of which are important to hernial therapy.

O) Like nearly every area of hernia science, there are differing opinions as to whether one should wear a hernia belt while exercising when supine and prone. Experiment, and/or consult your doctor, to determine what is best for you.

P) Feel free to change and adapt my exercises to whatever suits you. In fact, I encourage this. A physical fitness trainer can help you fine-tune these, and other abdomen building exercises (there are many to choose from), to fit your hernia therapeutic needs.

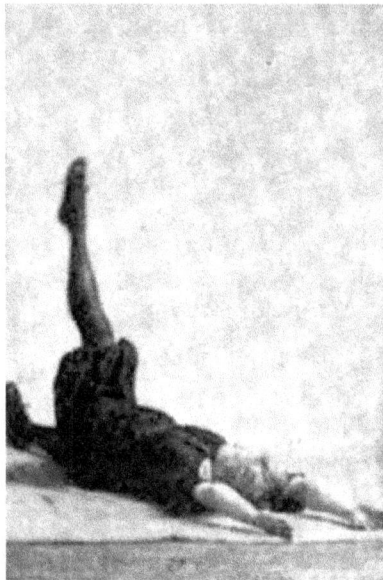

When it comes to healing an inguinal hernia, leg lifts, like those demonstrated here, are extremely important. The legs can be lifted singly or together.

THE EXERCISES
(One session, comprising 10 exercises, lasts approximately 15 minutes)

WARMUPS
EXERCISE 1: THE LEG LIFT
Lay flat on your back, face upward, with your legs straight out and your feet 1-2 feet apart (the supine position). Place your arms wherever they are most comfortable, usually with your hands about 1-2 feet from the body. (If you have back sensitivity, bend your knees, placing your feet flat on the floor.) Engage your core. Raise your right leg horizontally. Slowly lift and lower your leg 5-10 times without letting it touch the floor. After the last lift, hold your leg horizontally for 5 seconds. Rest. Repeat with the left leg.

EXERCISE 2: THE KNEE BEND
Assume the supine position described in Exercise 1. Engage your core. Slowly raise your right knee up toward your chest, then straighten your leg out again without touching the floor. Repeat 5-10 times. After the last knee bend, hold your leg horizontally for 5 seconds. Rest. Repeat with the left leg.

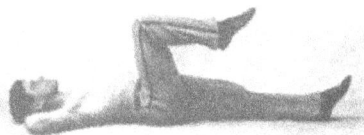

The Knee Bend.

EXERCISE 3: THE STRAIGHT LINE
Assume the supine position described in Exercise 1. Engage your core. Raise your right leg. Point your toes and slowly move your leg horizontally from left to right in a straight line 5-10 times. Do not let it touch the floor. After the last sweep, hold your leg horizontally for 5 seconds. Rest. Repeat with the left leg.

STRENGTHENING
EXERCISE 4: THE CIRCLE
Circle Exercise.

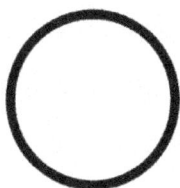

Assume the supine position described in Exercise 1. Engage your core. Raise your right leg. Point your toes and, moving clockwise, slowly draw a small imaginary circle (about 1 foot or so in diameter) in the air without letting your foot touch the floor. Do this 2-5 times. After the last circle, hold your leg horizontally for 5 seconds. Rest. Repeat with the left leg. Rest. Repeat with the right leg again, this time moving it in a counterclockwise direction. Rest. Repeat with the left leg moving in a counterclockwise direction.

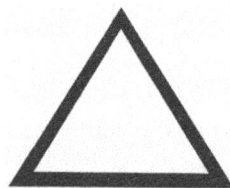

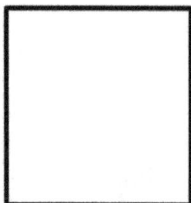

EXERCISE 5: THE TRIANGLE

Assume the supine position described in Exercise 1. Engage your core. Raise your right leg. Point your toes and, moving clockwise, slowly draw a large imaginary triangle in the air (with the tip at the top), without letting your foot touch the floor. Do this 2-5 times. After the last triangle, hold your leg horizontally for 5 seconds. Rest. Repeat with the left leg. Rest. Repeat with the right leg again, this time moving in a counterclockwise direction. Rest. Repeat with the left leg moving in a counterclockwise direction.

Triangle Exercise.

EXERCISE 6: THE SQUARE

Assume the supine position described in Exercise 1. Engage your core. Raise your right leg. Point your toes and, moving clockwise, slowly draw a large imaginary square in the air without letting your foot touch the floor. Do this 2-5 times. After the last square, hold your leg horizontally for 5 seconds. Rest. Repeat with the left leg. Rest. Repeat with the right leg again, this time moving in a counterclockwise direction. Rest. Repeat with the left leg moving in a counterclockwise direction.

Square Exercise.

TONING

EXERCISE 7: THE FROG KICK

Assume the supine position described in Exercise 1. Engage your core. Raise your right leg. Point your toes. Then, drawing your knee up toward your chest, slowly kick out, bringing your leg down and around again for another kick. Do this 5-10 times. After the last kick, hold your leg horizontally for 5 seconds. Rest. Repeat with the left leg. Rest. Repeat again with the right leg, this time moving in the opposite direction (that is, a reverse frog kick). Rest. Repeat again with the left leg moving in the opposite direction (reverse frog kick).

EXERCISE 8: THE BIRD DOG
Kneel on all fours with your palms flat on the floor. Engage your core. Hold out your left arm horizontally, then straighten out your right leg horizontally and slowly raise and lower it 5-10 times. After the last lift, hold your right leg horizontally for 5 seconds. Do the same with the right arm and the left leg.

ALTERNATE EXERCISE 8: THE EASY BIRD DOG
This is a less difficult version of the Bird Dog. Kneel on all fours with your palms flat on the floor. Engage your core. While keeping your palms on the floor, lift up and straighten out your right leg horizontally, then slowly raise and lower it 5-10 times. After the last lift, hold your right leg horizontally for 5 seconds. Place it back in a kneeling position. Do the same with the left leg.

EXERCISE 9: THE PLANK
Lay on your stomach. Engage your core. Raise yourself so that you are holding your entire body up off the floor on your palms (or fists) and toes. Maintain your head in a relaxed manner and facing the floor. Straighten out your back to a horizontal plank-like position. Hold this pose for 10-30 seconds. Rest on the floor. Repeat two more times. This is one of the best exercises for strengthening the muscles of the abdominal region, and also the back region.

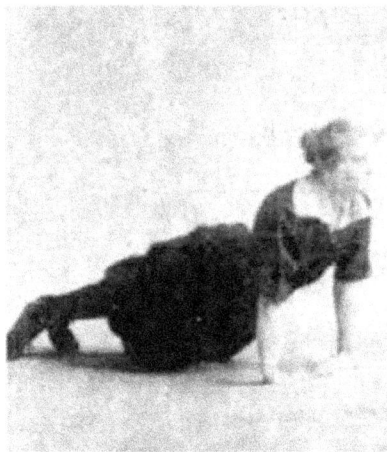

Victorian version of the plank. (Note: Some modern authorities do not recommend the plank for inguinal hernia.)

ALTERNATE EXERCISE 9: THE EASY PLANK
This is a less difficult version of the Plank. Lay on your stomach. Engage your core. Raise yourself so that you are holding yourself up off the floor on your forearms and bent knees. (Your forearms should be pointed forward and lined up directly under your shoulders. Your lower legs should be pointed upward at about a 45 degree angle behind you.) Straighten out your back to a horizontal plank-like position. Hold this pose for 10-30 seconds. Rest on the floor. Repeat two more times.

EXERCISE 10: THE SOCCER BALL KNEE SQUEEZE

Lay on your back. Bend your knees, placing your feet flat on the floor. Engage your core. Take a soccer ball (football in the UK) or a soccer ball size ball (one preferably made of soft rubber) and place it between your knees. Squeeze gently but firmly for 30-60 seconds. Repeat this 2-4 times. Excellent for strengthening the muscles around the inguinal canal.

END OF THE EXERCISES

HEALING TIME

If you do this workout correctly and regularly (1-2 times daily, for instance, morning and evening), you should begin to see small positive changes in your hernial condition within the first week or so, perhaps even in the first few days. By this I mean that your hernia should protrude less and less. The whole inguinal area should begin to feel more solid, muscular, and supportive with the passage of time. If you do not experience any overt or even subtle changes at first, do not lose hope. Stick to it (with your doctor's approval).

As some Victorian naturopaths reported, using a combination of truss and exercise, it is possible to cure an inguinal hernia in as little as 2 months.[176] On the other hand, more conservative 19th-Century doctors suggested allowing at least 6 months for a total hernia healing after beginning your "gymnastic" workouts.[177]

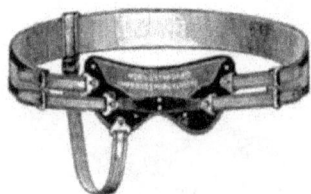

Victorian double elastic truss with elliptic spring on front plate.

The reality is that, depending on many variables (age, health, mental attitude, adherence to the hernia repair plan, etc.), your own cure period will probably range somewhere between 2 months and 6 months. However, the length of time it takes for a full healing is not as important as your commitment to persevere with your program, in particular your exercises (whatever program you choose or create for yourself).

Also bear in mind that, generally speaking, the longer you have had your hernia, the longer your body will need to heal itself. Be patient. Give Nature the time it needs to "work her magic."

As discussed, your body's natural state is health. It does not seek or want a reducible inguinal hernia, and it will eliminate it for you if provided with the proper means: correct hernia belt, correct fit, correct diet, correct posture, correct weight, correct attitude, and correct exercise. These practices, along with your daily abdominal exercise routine, must be kept up permanently if you wish to prevent the return of your inguinal hernia—or the emergence of a new one. Authentic full body-mind health requires a lifelong commitment.

The reward is potentially great for those willing to adhere to their chosen program. Eventually, you will find yourself needing to wear your hernia belt less and less. One day, if all goes well and your healing is accomplished, you should be able to discontinue its use completely. This is, after all, our ultimate goal, as Victorian healthcare professional Dr. Bilz noted in 1898:

☛ **As soon as the treatment shows satisfactory results the truss may now and again be removed . . . and gradually be left off all together.**[178]

NO GUARANTEES
Bear in mind that though my ultimate goal in resuscitating the hernia healing methods of the Victorian Period is to help you do away with your hernia belt altogether, there are never any guarantees. Not even your personal physician can guarantee a result.

However, if you follow his or her instructions in combination with the suggestions offered in this book, you will be well on your way to achieving your hernia goals.

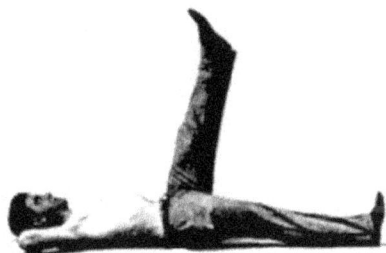

Hard work, belief, and perseverance tend to pay off. Goal achievement is not up to your family, friends, or doctor. It is up to you.

WHEN TO START
Victorian physicians were unified on at least one point: The sooner you begin your natural healing regimen the better. According to these particular sources, the longer you wait, the more difficult it may become to effect a cure. This is because, as Dr. Gour states earlier in this book:

☛ **A hernia that has been reducible may in time become irreducible because of adhesions, because of the growth** of omental fat, or because of the increase in size of the mass. It may result in serious complications because of its prominence, which renders it liable to bruise and thus give pain, or there is always danger of obstruction and strangulation. Irreducible hernia usually requires surgery.[179]

Despite Dr. Gour's pronouncement, the medical reality is that even hernias over one to two decades old can be and have been cured using natural methods—a fact clearly demonstrated by the case studies chronicled in Appendix A.

This does not, however, negate the good doctor's statement. It is always best to get on a healing program for your reducible inguinal hernia as soon as possible, since this decreases the opportunity for complications to arise while helping increase the odds of success. Let us recall Dr. Foote's advice from Chapter Two:

☞ The individual so affected, male or female, should then lose no time in adopting means for their cure, for unless they are at least protected by a good truss, they may at any moment assume a dangerous form and imperil the life of the sufferer.[180]

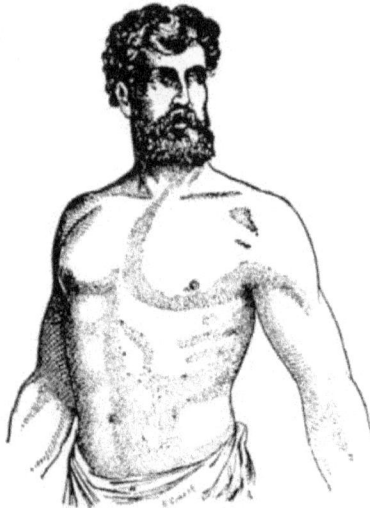

A healthy mind in a healthy body will always be the best preventative of and the best remedy for inguinal hernia.

SUMMARY

Combining the use of a well fitting hernia belt with the proper exercises, posture, diet, and mental attitude can achieve remarkable results, and the information I have provided here substantiates it.

I had a reducible inguinal hernia for many years, during which time I did the research that later became the subject of this book. I carefully followed the advice of Victorian doctors, as well as my own knowledge and intuition, and in two months my hernia was nearly gone. At the end of three months it had entirely disappeared and I am now truss-free. Thousands of others, both Victorian and modern, have shared similar testimonies.

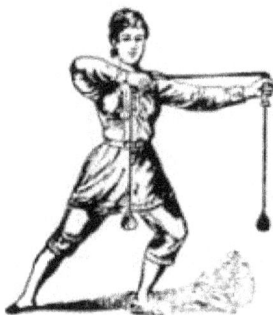

Victorian woman performing an abdomen-strengthening exercise, excellent for inguinal hernia.

You too can create your own miracle. But only if you are willing to educate yourself, work hard, make the necessary sacrifices, and devote yourself fully to the end goal. When Dr. Bilz's natural health program was criticized for being "troublesome" and requiring too "much labour," he replied:

☛ **Health is worth working for. It is very convenient to take medicine, and very easy to die. A few drops of prussic acid are enough to kill a patient in five minutes, but long years of labour are required to restore him to health. Which of the two would the wise man choose?**[181]

Remember: While advice and assistance are readily available to you from a myriad of sources, in the end it is you and your immune system alone that must do all of the real work.

Godspeed. Get busy.

THE END

EXERCISE

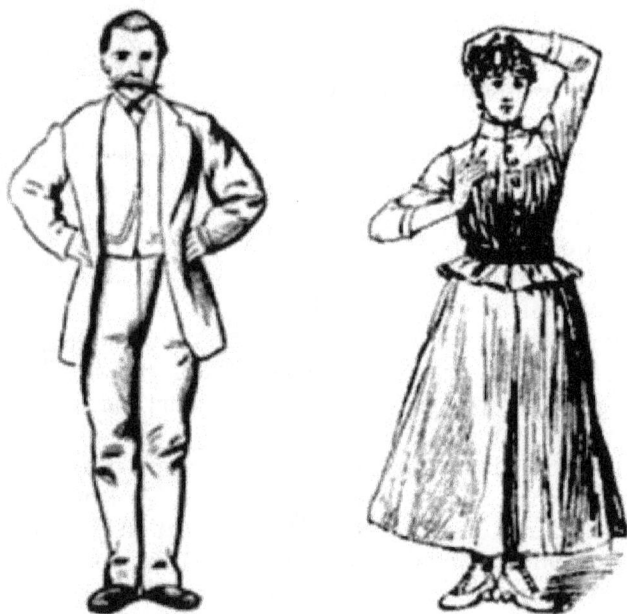

Keep at it!

APPENDIX A
Fifteen Cases of Naturally Healed Hernias

W hat follows is documentation of naturally cured hernias (of various types, some after failed surgeries) by the Victorian English surgeon Dr. William Dufour and his London clinic, the "Institution for the Radical Cure of Rupture and of Stricture." I have excerpted this material from his 1821 book, *A Treatise on the Radical Cure of Hernia or Rupture*. Since his patients were treated 201 years ago, I of course cannot vouch for the legitimacy of the doctor's testimonials. The reader may make of them what he or she will. Assuming they are genuine, they are not only impressive, they correlate with my own personal hernia healing experience as well as thousands of others.

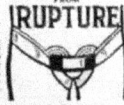

A Victorian truss ad from *Confederate Veteran* magazine. It promises "rupture sufferers" that this "appliance" will "bind and draw the broken parts together."

The cases are arranged by Dr. Dufour according to age, the youngest first. He writes:

> **"By this arrangement, those afflicted with rupture will be the better enabled to perceive that the time of life, late or early, opposes no effectual obstacle to the success of our efforts. Infancy, prime manhood, middle age, the decline of life, nay its very extremity have alike presented us with opportunities for trying our remedy, and at all those periods of human existence has our remedy, succeeded."**

For understandable reasons at the time (1821), Dr. Dufour did not reveal the details of his then "newly discovered treatment" for inguinal hernia. It is safe to say, however, that it was something similar to the nonsurgical remedy that I and the naturopathic doctors in this very book suggest: a combination of exercise, diet, and hernia belt; probably with an assortment of other therapies, such as massage, herbs, acupuncture, baths, etc. These were the standard healing modalities in the school of Victorian naturopathy.

More importantly to our topic, these 19th-Century health regimens have not become obsolete merely because they are now rejected and ridiculed by the majority of modern conventional medical practitioners. They are as relevant and curative today as they were in the 1900s, and the sagacious will consider them as such.

Before reading the following successful case studies, please note the full title of Dr. Dufour's book:

A Treatise on the Radical Cure of Hernia or Rupture, Effected Without any Surgical Operation, Pain, or Suspension of the Patient's Ordinary Avocations

ᛦᚻE ᛦᚪSES

Mr. S. M. Aged 22

☞ 1. This gentleman had experienced during five years, all the inconveniences attending inguinal rupture, or rupture appearing at the right groin. His spirits had become unusually depressed, and, until his application to us for relief, such was his state of mind, that business of every kind distressed him, and his professional duties remained entirely undischarged. From the day our remedy was first applied he gradually improved in health and strength; with them, of course, were assumed his more grateful mental feelings; in about ten weeks every symptom of rupture had ceased and he was therefore pronounced cured.[182]

Miss M. R. Aged 24

☞ 2. This was also a case of inguinal rupture; but it appeared at the left groin. The symptoms and appearances except in point of duration, were scarcely distinguishable from the last case. There was indeed somewhat greater disarrangement of the general health, which the patient attributed to the disorder; and the justness of this presumed foundation became verified, by reason that with the gradual recession of the intestine within its proper bounds, her health and spirits took their natural and grateful tone. The cure was in progress eight weeks, and then effected without the patient having experienced pain or inconvenience from the treatment.[183]

Mr. T. B. Aged 26

☞ 3. This was a case of scrotal rupture descending from the right side. It had existed somewhat more than seven years. It had at times been extremely painful, and latterly had considerable influence upon the spirits. Loss of appetite and consequent debility had quite incapacitated him from attending to his ordinary concerns. In trusses it appears Mr. B. did not place any confidence; and never having used one, although the rupture had been so longstanding, he applied to us. Amendment soon began to be visible, yet the case did not terminate in cure, till after about two months persevering treatment. At the expiration of that time Mr. B. was cured. In this patient, both during and previously to the application of our remedies the degree of mental depression was very great. But in this as in many other cases of rupture and consequent mental depression, the spirits rose as the disease gave way, and Mr. B. is now perfectly well and sound.[184]

Miss S. B. Aged 27

☞ 4. This was a case of inguinal rupture, that is to say of rupture appearing at the left groin. So formidable had it been, as once to have put the young lady's life in extreme hazard. The disease previously to its being submitted to our care, had been standing eight years, and about a year after it first became visible, local pain, at intervals more or less distant from each other occurred. At length the family as well as the young lady were alarmed on learning from the surgeon who was consulted, that all the terrific symptoms which were then present, arose from the rupture having become strangulated. It would be useless to enlarge upon the agony experienced by Miss B. . . . The Surgeon with great skill, proportioned to the difficulty of the case, succeeded in obviating the strangulation without operating. For six or seven succeeding years the disease remained stationary; not often or much affecting the young lady; yet the tumour was observed to be on the increase: and at length, the pains too well recollected not to be dreaded, began to return. Anticipation of what might happen became strengthened by what had, and the tumour still increasing, Miss B. was advised to put her case under our care. With singular patience Miss B. permitted the application of our remedies. They soon indicated the probability of early and complete success; and after eight weeks perseverance in the means of cure she was whole. It will have been obvious from the relation, of this case, that it was one of no ordinary nature; yet complete cure was at no period of our treatment doubtful. More than a year has elapsed since the cure was effected and now, not a vestige of the disease remains.[185]

Mr. J. P. Aged 34

☛ 5. This case exhibited a complete relaxation of the restraining powers of the belly. A double inguinal rupture, or rupture appearing at each groin. Originally of habits active; of strength adequate to a business rather laborious than requiring the utmost exertion of strength, and always with good appetite and of a cheerful disposition. But all these gave way, and diminished, as the disease increased. Two ruptures called early for surgical interposition, and almost immediately on their being observed, the application of a spring truss, presumed of strength sufficient to sustain both ruptures, was adopted. But it was unavailing; the pressure of the truss was great; but still the ruptures protruded from beneath the bulbs or pads. When this occurred which it frequently did, Mr. P. experienced very considerable pain. That pain would be felt in no slight degree upon such occasions will be obvious. A strong spring, pressing a soft or yielding body against a hard unyielding bone must necessarily create pain; yet Mr. P. went on for three years and a half, combating his double malady with trusses of every form and description; but the Ruptures increasing considerably in size, he began to apprehend himself to be in more than ordinary danger, and at length placed himself under our care. The case was not without its difficulties. The previous perseverance from year to year in the use of trusses, of various and generally of increased pressure, had interposed obstacles in the way of successful treatment. And in this case, we cannot say that the cure was effected without some inconvenience being felt by the patient. Our conjoint perseverance at length prevailed, but not until after ten weeks struggle against the magnitude of the disease. The parts affected have retired within their proper limits; there they remain, and Mr. P. is again whole and sound.[186]

Major B. Aged 36

☞ 6. This case was scrotal; the protrusion from the left side. It was remarkable for its duration, having subsisted for eighteen years. A truss had been applied as early as the disease had become visible; its use had not on any occasion been suspended; but no favourable alteration of the rupture had followed. The rupture could not be traced to any certain origin. Our inquiries as to the origin of individual cases of rupture have seldom been successful. It is probably too much connected with the general habits of the patient, and therefore the very identical or proximate cause, will not easily have been perceived by him. In all likelihood in this, as in most other cases, the descent of the intestine had been gradual. This gentleman had not been exposed to any very great inconvenience from his rupture. Yet riding and, indeed, every little exertion beyond his ordinary foot exercise, gave him somewhat more than sensation; not quite perhaps amounting to pain: or if pain it were, it was only just sufficient to remind him that exercise should not be pushed too far. Yet the major determined to submit his case to our treatment, and in less than eight weeks his cure was happily and completely effected.[187]

Mr. J. E. Aged 36

☞ 7. This was a case of femoral rupture; or of rupture below the groin, at the bend of the right thigh. The disease had been of three years standing. A truss applied in its most early stages, had not in the slightest degree apparently checked its progress. The tumour had increased so very considerably in size, as to impede walking. Mr. E. had from time to time suffered all the symptoms of his disease, short indeed of those where strangulation takes place, but sufficiently harrassing and even distressing of themselves to occasion depression of spirits, loss of appetite and of strength. He at length submitted his case to our inspection. The tumour just at the bend of the thigh measured more than three inches over. Except in this respect, Mr. E's case was unattended with any symptom not common to most cases of rupture. This gentleman remained under our care above eleven weeks, and at the expiration of that period, had become completely whole and sound; not a trace of rupture remaining.[188]

Mr. J. R. Aged 37

☞ 8. This was also a case of double inguinal rupture; or of rupture appearing at both groins. The patient had been engaged in the sea service, which service the length and augmenting severity of his disease had obliged him to quit. The tumours had existed nine years, and at the time the treatment of the case was undertaken by us, they were manifestly on the increase. With their size, pain and inconvenience increased also, attended with loss of appetite and great prostration of strength. From Mr. R's account of his case, this last symptom was very remarkable. Our course of treatment continued about eleven weeks, and we participated in the patients feelings, consequent upon the gradual restoration of his more healthy and more grateful state; his appetite soon improved; his strength returned: and at the expiration of that time his disease was no longer to be perceived. . . .[189]

Mr. J. W. Aged 38

☛ 9. This was a case of inguinal rupture; or of rupture appearing at the right groin. It had been standing five years, and twice in the course of that space of time had his life been in hazard from the rupture having become strangulated. On both those dreadful occasions the patient had been relieved by surgical aid. The patient's general health had much suffered and any degree of increased exertion, no matter how small, occasioned considerable pain in the part affected. He at length placed himself under our care, and after ten weeks perseverance our treatment terminated in complete cure.[190]

Mrs. M. A. Aged 47

☛ 10. This was a case of umbilical rupture; or of rupture appearing at the navel. On the case being first submitted to our care, the tumour at the navel was large and circumscribed. Its nature could not be mistaken. The symptoms were occasional pain at the part and general in disposition, not easily referable to any cause other than that of local mischief. The complaint had been standing about three years; for a great part of which time a truss, adapted to the part had been worn; from its application, no apparent good, farther than some corroboration had resulted, and Mrs. A. at length consulted us. In about two months, progress towards cure had become very evident, and our treatment terminated in that most desirable event in ten weeks from the first application of our remedies.[191]

Mr. S. Aged 48

☛ 11. This was a case of inguinal rupture; or of rupture appearing at the right groin; of three years standing. The patient had not worn a truss, and at the time the case came first under our notice, the tumour was quite unequivocal in its appearance; it was large, and Mr. S. complained of occasionally suffering much pain in the part. Motion of the right thigh had become inconvenient; and general debility was to him a source of considerable despondence. The pain and other common symptoms of the disease became, at length, even upon slight exercise much aggravated. He at length submitted himself to our care; amendment soon became visible, and his complete cure was effected in eleven weeks.[192]

Mr. A. Aged 48

☛ 12. This was also a case of inguinal rupture, or of rupture appearing at the right groin; its duration had been three years and a half: during the whole of which space of time, attended with aggravated symptoms, and particularly with cough of the most harrassing description. A truss had been early applied, but from the violence of the cough, the truss rather prejudiced than protected the patient. On the accession of a coughing fit, the rupture would slide below the pad; and sharp pain occasioned by the consequent pressure took place in this case as already related in that of Mr. J. P. This pain was only relievable by removing the truss, by reducing the part protruded and by again subjecting the rupture to less unequal pressure. That the cough and rupture mutually acted upon each other and reciprocally distressed the patient, there cannot be a doubt; for the progress of the cure of the rupture, was marked most gratefully to the patient by a gradual diminution of the cough. Other distressing symptoms were, an oppressive sense of weight at the lower part of the belly, and, generally, extreme lassitude. After treating the case about nine weeks, a complete cure was effected.[193]

Mr. W. T. Aged 50

☛ 13. This was a case of a very aggravated description; a double rupture, but appearing at different points; that is to say, inguinal, or at the left groin; and scrotal, descending from the right side of the lower belly. These ruptures having no assignable cause within the patient's recollection, had existed only about eight months; but their progress from the first, although attempted to be restrained by a truss, was very rapid. The application of the truss was attended with no beneficial result whatever. The scrotal rupture was at times attended with much inflammation and pain; the size of both ruptures became alarming, and the going up and down stairs was impracticable without extreme torture. The patient was compelled therefore to dwell upon the ground floor of his house, and at the time he submitted his case to our notice, all the aforementioned evils had increased. The treatment was in point of time necessarily protracted; but a beneficial termination was always anticipated: and in three months the cure was completed.[194]

Mr. I. Aged 51

☛ 14. This was a case of inguinal rupture, or of rupture appearing at the right groin. It had been standing seventeen years, but from the first a truss had been applied, the benefit derived from which for the first fourteen years, was merely negative. During the last three years, the truss had appeared wanting in its presumed efficacy, and the tumour had in that space of time very much increased. With the increase of size considerable pain was also felt in the part; and any sort of exertion, was attended with more or less inconvenience. Latterly the truss had been worse than useless, the rupture frequently slipping from beneath the pad. From the partial pressure thereby occasioned, the pain became much augmented, and the patient began to anticipate danger. This gentleman had from the commencement of his disease been extremely nice and scrupulous both as to the forms of his trusses, for he tried many, and in endeavouring to keep them exactly applied to the part affected. His case, finally, became subjected to our treatment, and although the cure was much impeded by the continuance of a severe constitutional cough, a cure was completely effected in the space of fifteen weeks.[195]

The Right Honourable the Earl of _____. Aged 78
☛ 15. This nobleman had been ruptured fifteen years. The disease was inguinal, appearing at the right groin. It was attended with no one alarming symptom, yet the rupture was sufficiently distinct. Slight pain indeed, now and then occurred, which, conscious of his disorder, his lordship, conceived might thence originate. Apprehending the possibility of further mischief his lordship was induced to honour us with his confidence; and in about fourteen weeks, had the gratification of seeing his cure complete, not a vestige of his disease remaining. The remarkable features in this case, were the great age of the noble patient, and the duration of the disease. His lordship has with singular urbanity been graciously pleased to sanction a personal reference for the authenticity of this cure. But while we most respectfully solicited this liberty, we pledged ourselves that the occasion would be particular indeed, which should influence us to trouble his lordship.[196]

> In the foregoing cases, numerous and authentic as they are, we have taken upon ourselves briefly and candidly without the slightest exaggeration, to relate the facts incidental to them.[197] — William Dufour (1821)

A magazine ad from 1923.

"It is a surer method, more fruitful of results, and more worthy of a man, to develop and to earn health as far as possible by personal activity, than when it is lost to look passively to nature, or to drugs to bring about its slow return."

Daniel Gottlieb Moritz Schreber, 1899

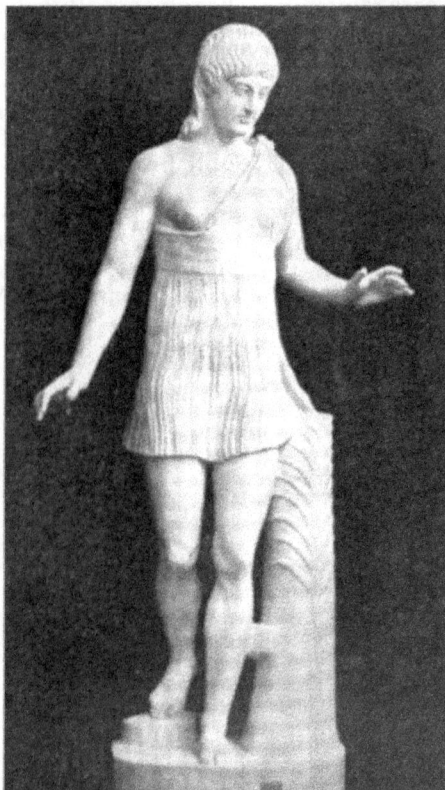

This 5'11" marble statue of an ancient European "girl runner," housed at Rome's Vatican Museum, is a copy of an original bronze that dates from around 470 B.C. The 14 year old Dorian female depicted—possibly a victress from one of the girls' games held at Sparta or Rome—symbolizes the ardent devotion to physical fitness and health that was common in ancient Roman and Greek culture. Writes Walter W. Hyde in 1921: "While excluded from the [Olympic] games proper, women had their own festival at Olympia in honor of [the goddess] Hera, which was known as the *Heraia*. These games occurred every four years and included a foot-race . . . in which the course was one-sixth less than the stadion. The victress received an olive crown and also a share of the cow sacrificed to Hera, and was allowed to set up a painted picture of herself in the Heraion." Our modern Olympic Flame was borrowed from the ancient tradition of burning a continuous torch on Hera's altar during the games.

APPENDIX B
The Truss in Hernia Healing

The following essay is from Dr. Edward B. Foote's 1864 book *Medical Common Sense*. While most of it may seem like a sponsored ad for a then popular 19th-Century hernia product (known commercially as "Hicks' Air-Inflated Rubber Truss Pads"), I have included it here for the valuable information it contains on self-healing, which may assist and inspire my more inventive readers:

☞ Not many years have elapsed since it was thought by medical men that external, no less than internal rupture, and hernia were incurable; that all that could be done, was to retain the contents of the sac within their proper walls by a well adjusted truss. In process of time, however, it was found that irritation or inflammation of the parts induced by uncomfortable and badly fitted pads, in rare instances, caused an adhesion of the ruptured membranes or a contraction of the relaxed apertures and canals, and the patient became relieved of his troublesome affection. This fact led some doctors to believe that they could get up this adhesive inflammation by surgical operations, and success attended their experiments so far as the production of the inflammation was concerned; but, unfortunately, they found it difficult to control it, and their patients oftener died than recovered, with inflammation in the peritoneum. Such operations are occasionally performed now, but they are extremely hazardous, and no one who does not wish to run the risk of sudden death, should submit to such experimenting.

After the "heroic doctors" had tried their hands till it seemed that death rather than recovery followed their dangerous operations, some enterprising truss establishments undertook to introduce trusses, the pads of which were so arranged as to press on the rupture or hernia with so much severity as to induce this adhesive inflammation in many cases. This was a partial success, but so far as my observation enabled me to judge, the victims of these expedients were almost punched out of the world, such was the pressure required to produce the desired adhesive inflammation. These contrivances are somewhat employed now, but the public has become pretty much disgusted with them, and they will eventually, like old almanacs, become entirely obsolete.

Science moves on, unless bound with the chains of old fogyism, and unsuccessful inventions often suggest to ingenious minds those which do prove a triumph. Progress has been made in the invention and manufacture of pads to cure rupture and hernia. Dr. [Lucien E.] Hicks, in 1855, invented an inflated rubber pad, which, though never advertised nor brought prominently before the public, became very popular and called forth the highest recommendation from the celebrated Prof. [Benjamin] Silliman of Yale College, and from other scientific men, among whom were eminent surgeons. It was not claimed for this pad that it would effect cures, but its comfortable elasticity, cleanliness, etc., gave it the precedence as a comfortable appliance, and from this circumstance it was popularly denominated the "relief pad." Notwithstanding the modest claims for it, however, it effected many cures. This was, no doubt, in consequence of its not interfering with nature's curative operations when she was disposed to remedy the difficulty herself, for *there can be no question that both rupture and hernia would often be restored by the natural healing process* [my emphasis, L.S.] if not prevented by a hard unyielding truss-pad, which aggravates the difficulty rather than aids in its cure.

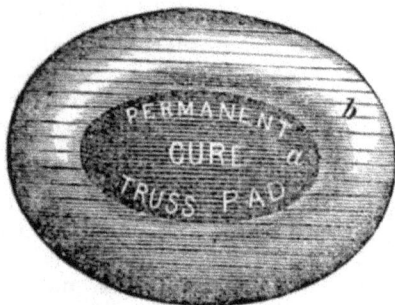

Top view of the Permanent Cure Pad, 1864. Parts: a) The oval naked rubber ball in the center for exciting the adhesive inflammation; b) the cloth-covered rubber ring cushion.

The success of the relief pad subsequently led the inventor to introduce a companion for it, which he named the "Permanent Cure Pad." Every one who has ever worn an unlined india-rubber shoe for a little while, next [to] the skin of the foot, knows full well how tender and sore the flesh becomes. The naked rubber seems to have a drawing and irritating effect when applied for a length of time to any portion of the human body, and soreness and tenderness indicating the presence of inflammation ensue. From this fact Dr. H. drew the very philosophical conclusion that a [softer] pad ... would, without the discomfort and uncertainty attending the application of hard pads with a painful pressure, produce the necessary adhesive inflammation. [His invention uses] .. . an oblong ball of naked rubber [that] protrudes from the center. Even this ball is inflated with air, as well as the ring which surrounds it, so that its pressure is not painful nor irritating to the outer skin. Indeed, the pressure is not greatly unlike that of the ball of the finger when pressed gently upon the part, and the adhesive inflammation it induces is produced entirely by the properties of the rubber before explained.

The application of the permanent cure pad, until soreness is induced, followed by the relief pad, to sustain the contents of the rupture or hernia while the healing process is going on, has thus far proved a perfect success in all cases not confirmed by age, and in many long standing cases of persons quite advanced in life, it has proved remarkably and gratifyingly successful. Nor does the inflammation induced by the permanent cure pads seem to involve the peritoneum in the least. No case has occurred in which any troublesome or fatal results have followed their use. The patient has only to apply the pads and effect for himself the cure without any danger whatever. The merits of both the permanent cure and relief pads may be briefly summed up as follows:

1st. They are not expensive. Various contrivances of an uncertain and painful nature for the radical cure of hernia have been offered to the afflicted, but the charge for such appliances has been usually from twenty to thirty dollars, whereas the permanent cure pad and the relief pad of this description are furnished at incomparably lower prices.

2nd. They are elastic. While they possess sufficient resistance to retain the most troublesome hernia, they readily yield to every motion of the body, whether natural, as in walking or in other exercise, or convulsive, as in sneezing, coughing, laughing, etc. It is well known that stuffed pads become matted and unyielding, and that wooden or porcelain pads are from the first moment of their adjustment uncomfortable. One might as well be punched in the abdomen with a stick, as to cough or sneeze with one of those unelastic contrivances attached to his person. It is found, too, that such an unyielding pressure on the parts, interferes not only with the circulation of the blood, but with the healthy distribution of the nervous forces, and paralysis of the parts not unfrequently ensues. Those who have long worn ordinary truss pads need no argument to convince them of the truthfulness of this remark.

3rd. They will not shift from the part to which they are properly adjusted. Their elasticity causes them to so conform to the anatomy of the parts to which they are applied, that any motion of the body does not disturb their position. This is no mere theory. Those who have worn them, uniformly testify to their possession of this virtue. The wearer may lift, jump, run, sneeze, etc., without changing their position above, or below the ruptured or relaxed aperture, which fact proves them to be constant protectors against protrusions of hernia, under any circumstances.

4th. They are cleanly. The perspiration will not penetrate the rubber, while the sweaty secretions are readily carried off by the cloth covering the surface of the relief pad, and nearly covering that of the permanent cure pad. Then too they can be readily removed from their metallic attachment. They may then be washed with soap and water, and dried in five minutes. This is an important consideration for those who wear hard pads, for cleanliness. The readiness with which the pad can be removed from the metallic plate which attaches it to the truss, also makes it convenient for changing the pads when desired. Thus the permanent cure pad can be removed, and the relief pad substituted in a moment by any person.

5th. They are durable. They will remain in good order a life-time for those afflicted with incurable ruptures. A more significant proof of the truthfulness of this claim is not needed than the fact that a large truss establishment in this city, objected to the adoption of the pad in its trade, on the ground only, that it would never wear out! The proprietors seemed to fear that such a durable pad would injure the business.

6th. The metallic attachment is such that a patient may wear an oscillating, or a fast pad, as preferred. Some prefer what is commonly called "ball and socket," while others will only have a firmly fastened pad. By removing the screws, which anyone can do with his fingers from the bulb on the underside of the brass plate, the pad will oscillate without obstruction. Those wishing a fast pad, by adjusting the screws with a screw-driver, or knife-blade, can set it firmly at any angle desired. Those who have never worn a truss, can with this pad choose between an oscillating and a firm one, by trying both without extra expense.

7th. The pad may be attached to any truss which the wearer may now be using. In a majority of cases it may be done by the patient him or herself, but if not, any mechanic, even a blacksmith, can make an attachment in a few minutes, and at an expense not to exceed twenty-five cents. This is a valuable feature for any one who presently possesses a good spring, and only desires to adopt these valuable pads, or who, living at a distance, wishes to be fitted to a spring at home, and have these pads put on.

Thus in brief I have named the chief merits of the Hicks pads, which any intelligent person must perceive will eventually take the place of all others now before the public. They must commend themselves to every one, and all who have not tested their utility, may well reason that if the relief pad as formerly constructed, called forth the recommendation of

Side view of the Permanent Cure Pad, showing: a) ball; b) corrugated cloth pad; c) plate attachment ledge; d) spring receiver where pad is attached to the truss.

Prof. Silliman after eighteen months' experience and observation, for not only its comfortableness but its liability to effect cures, the use of both the permanent cure pad and the relief pad, cannot fail to effect all that is claimed for them, and the claim is simply this: *that in all cases of reducible rupture and hernia in which a cure is possible, the wearing of the permanent cure pad, followed by the application, for a time, of the relief pad, will unite the walls through which the bowel or any part protrudes, and restore the ruptured or enlarged apertures or canals to their former healthy condition, thereby rendering all truss appliances unnecessary, even for protection.* Thousands of cases supposed to be incurable, may be permanently cured by this process, and at an expense far less than by any other method known to the profession or public. Although less expensive, they will do more toward effecting a cure than any other appliances in use.

Before concluding this essay, a few hints as to the most effective means resorted to for the reduction of hernia when reducible, may be properly introduced, inasmuch as such advice may enable the non-professional reader to attend to a case of this kind, when the services of an experienced surgeon cannot be easily obtained.

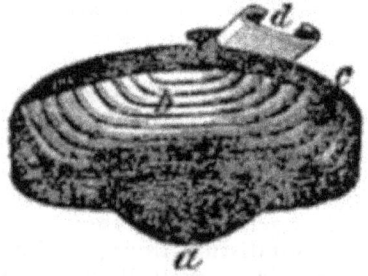

. . . In adults, the following methods may be generally successfully employed: The patient must be laid on his back with his head very low and his breech [buttocks] raised high with pillows. In this situation flannel cloths wrung out of a decoction of mallows or chamomile flowers, or even warm alone, are applied [to the hernia], and kept on the spot till the parts become sufficiently relaxed to allow the bowel [i.e., the herniated or protruding organ] to return. If this does not result in a little time, a clyster [enema] of this same decoction, with a large spoonful of butter and an ounce or two of common salt may be thrown up into the rectum by the anus or back passage of the body. The observance of these rules is often sufficient of itself, to return the hernia, but if they should not prove successful, recourse must then be had to pressure. If the tumor be very hard, a good degree of force will be required. Mere force, however, will not always succeed. The operator while making the pressure with the palm of his hand, must with his fingers so handle the gut as to artfully slip it in by the same aperture through which it first came out of the cavity of the abdomen. The good effects of these manipulations are greatly aided by watching the respiration or breathing of the patient, and only pressing the protrusion when the air is exhaled from the body, inasmuch as the inflation of the lungs produces more or less pressure on the bowels.

Clysters or enemas, better known as injections, are sometimes made of warm water and the smoke of tobacco, and prove entirely successful. As soon as the parts are returned, an appropriate truss should be put on, and if comfort and cure are desired, no pads can be employed equal to which latter is secured by the Hicks rubber air-inflated pads herein described.[198]

The following text by Dr. Foote provides additional information on the "Hicks' Air-Inflated Rubber Truss Pads" discussed by him above:

☛ [Concerning] . . . the nature and value of these excellent pads. . . I shall say very little in this place except to place on record the certificates of Prof. Benj. Silliman, of Yale College, and Dr. Valentine Mott, the well known surgeon:

"I consider the improved truss-pad of Dr. Lucien E. Hicks a very valuable addition to the means of protection, in cases to which trusses are applicable. Nothing is so elastic as air, with which the pad is filled, and the envelope of rubber in which it is included, furnishes the best security against its escape.

"The ratchet and spring enable the wearer to adjust the degree of pressure exactly to his own particular case, while the elasticity of the pad is very favorable to the closing of the ring through which the bowel is liable to protrude.

"The holes in the brass plate that covers the pad enable one to give it a position to the right or left, until by trial the proper inclination is ascertained.

"By this improved truss, if applied early, before the

[hernial] ring is too much enlarged, a cure may be effected, and a complete protection may in all cases be attained.

"The elasticity of the hoop must of course be ascertained by trial, and will be various in different cases. When the elasticity is of the proper degree, and the hoop is protected by appropriate stuffing under the strap, the truss of Dr. Hicks becomes a very comfortable appendage, and can be worn without any annoyance.

"The preceding observations are the result of a critical attention, during the last eighteen months, to different varieties and trials of this truss, and are now communicated for the benefit of the inventor and his representatives, and their patients." — B. SILLIMAN.

The celebrated surgeon Dr. Valentine Mott added his testimony as follows:

"I think the improved patent truss of Dr. L. E. Hicks, an excellent invention. The air-pad constitutes its greatest novelty and improvement." — VALENTINE MOTT, Prof. of Materia Medica and Surgery.

These pads may be obtained by mail by those at a distance, at no greater cost than if applied for personally at my office. The prices are as follows: One relief pad, three dollars; two relief pads, five dollars; one permanent cure pad, and one relief pad, five dollars; one permanent cure pad, and two relief pads, seven dollars. Sent by mail to all parts of the United States, postage paid, on the receipt of the price. They can be attached without difficulty, to any truss, so that any one who already possesses a good spring, has only to obtain the pads.

Persons sending cash orders by mail, will receive the pads promptly, postage prepaid, accompanied with all necessary directions for applying them.

In all cases desiring to obtain a radical cure, at least a pair of pads will be necessary, one permanent cure pad and one relief pad. After the former has produced the necessary adhesive inflammation, the relief pad should be put on, and worn until the parts become strong and healthy. Those having incurable hernia, will find no pad equal to the relief pad for comfort and durability.

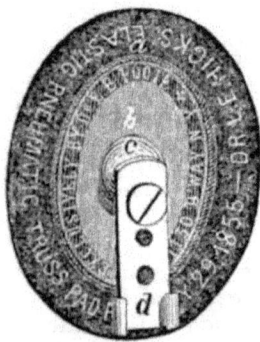

A back view of the Permanent Cure Pad, showing its: a) metal plate; b) the groove for attaching the plate; c) the ball socket; d) the spring receiver attachment.

Trusses with necessary pads complete, will be furnished in my office or by express for $10, except in cases of double rupture or hernia. A truss with all the necessary pads for the latter, is $15. In ordering by mail, measurements must be given. If there be but one rupture or hernia, the measure must be made from the tumor [hernia] in an opposite direction across the bowels, and around the hip on the opposite side from the tumor to the back-bone. This will be better understood when I inform the reader that the spring I furnish, does not go from the tumor around to the back on the same side on which the tumor protrudes, but comes from the back around the side opposite the tumor. In cases of double rupture or hernia, I must have the measurement around the body by placing the end of a piece of tape or tape-measure at the lowest extremity of the abdomen and passing it around the hips and body to the starting place.

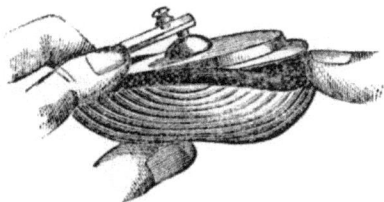

Disconnecting the pad from the metallic attachment.

Orders, whether for pads alone, or for a truss, must invariably be accompanied with the money according to the prices stated in the foregoing.

To the citizens of New York and vicinity: All of you who are afflicted with rupture or hernia are urgently requested to examine every variety of truss pads, and other appliances for the relief and cure of these difficulties within your knowledge, before examining these; for the rubber air pads which I offer challenge comparison, and only an examination of them is necessary to convince every one, that nothing has yet been discovered which can in any degree equal them.

Such is the verdict of all my professional acquaintances, of every surgeon to whom I have shown them, and of every patient who has worn them.

It is not expected that truss establishments will adopt these pads in their trade. They are altogether too durable. It is not for the interest of those who are wholly engaged in that department of trade and depending exclusively on it, to furnish goods which can hardly wear out. The inventor [Hicks] has intrusted their exclusive manufacture in my hands, and very likely those who need them will be unable to obtain them from any other source. I shall be glad to supply truss houses with them at prices that will allow first-rate profits to dealers, if they are willing to supply something which will either cure the patient or last him nearly his lifetime. My address will be found below.[199]

DR. E. B. FOOTE
May be consulted daily (except Sundays), between the hours of 1 and 7 P.M., at his Office and Residence, No. 1130 Broadway, New York City, between 25th and 26th streets (a few doors above the Fifth Avenue Hotel and nearly opposite the St. James.) His Summer Office at Saratoga Springs has been discontinued.[200]

HEALTH IS WEALTH

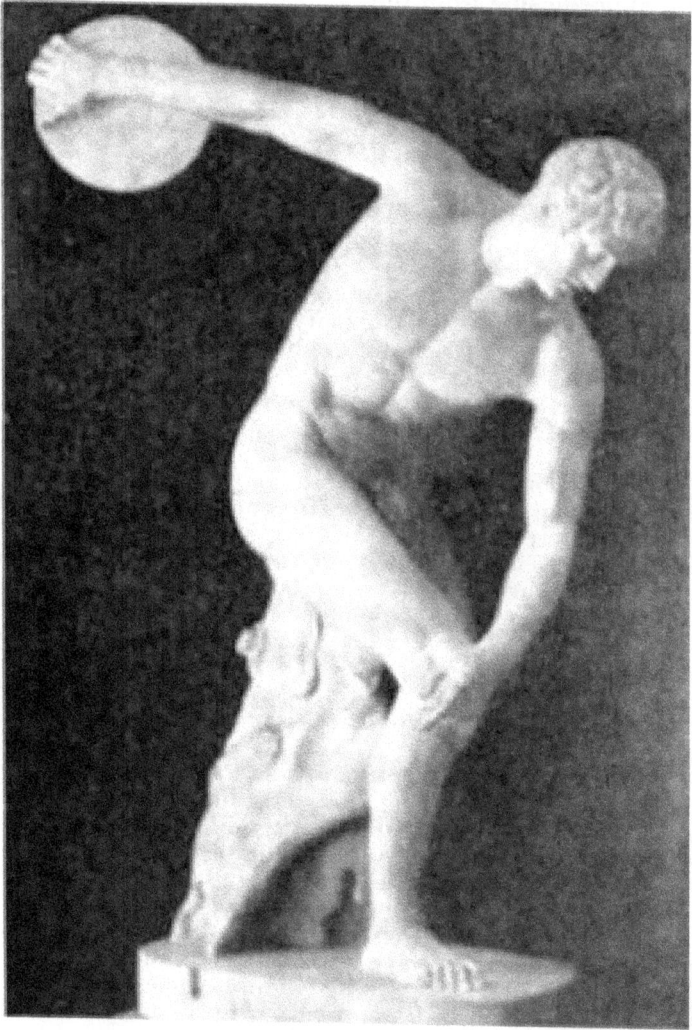

The *Diskobolos*, or Discus-thrower, a copy of the original by the noted ancient Athenian bronze-caster Myron (460 B.C. to 420 B.C.), "is perhaps the most famous athletic statue of all times." Despite the "violent exertions" often experienced by ancient Olympic athletes, like the one portrayed here, contrary to modern common wisdom, they seldom acquired inguinal hernias for the simple reason that they performed intense daily abdominal muscle exercises. As has been shown throughout this book, strong healthy abdominal musculature is one of the best safeguards against inguinal hernia. It has no replacement.

NOTES

1. Foote, p. 202. Some other interesting stats: During the Victorian Era most hernias occurred in people between the ages of 40 and 80. For obvious reasons, elderly women had the least. Concerning occupation, hernias were most common among male farmers, with wheelwrights having the least number of hernias. Finally, according to 19th-Century studies, most hernias occur on the right side of the body, while the individual most likely to experience a hernia was someone living in a warm climate. Warren, pp. 43-47. From a 1907 report: 96.3 percent of hernias in men are inguinal; 50.6 percent of hernias in women are inguinal. Eccles, p. 3.
2. Warren, pp. 43-44. Men and women with inguinal hernias make up a large percentage of patients at short-stay hospitals. See e.g., Haupt and Graves, p. 325.
3. Foote, p. 202; De Garmo, p. 18. The following list is of the most common hernias, beginning with inguinal (which comprises at least 75 percent of all hernias): inguinal, femoral, umbilical, ventral, obturator, sciatic, lumbral, perineal, vaginal, diaphragmatic. See Eccles, p. 2. Other types of hernia include: epigastric, hypochondriacal, ventral, crural, ischiatic, rectal, labial, scrotal, enteronal, invaginal, encysted, ligamentatic, diverticular. See Dowell, pp. 14-16.
4. *Pacific Medical Journal* (November 1893), p. 717.
5. *The Surgical Clinics of Chicago*, p. 21.
6. Edsall and Kent, p. 177.
7. *Annual Report of the Surgeon General, U.S. Navy, for the Fiscal Year 1926*, p. 207.
8. Pokras and Hufnagel, p. 3.
9. Website: www.fda.gov/medical-devices/implants-and-prosthetics/hernia-surgical-mesh-implants
10. See Hare, *PM*, pp. 40-42.
11. Tillmanns, p. 180.
12. For more on congenital inguinal hernia, see Keen and White, p. 912.
13. In 1900 Dr. William B. Eccles wrote: "A reducible hernia may be defined as one in which the contents of the sac can be returned to the abdomen. As a rule, the sac of a hernia is fixed to the surrounding tissue, and cannot be displaced except by dissection. Most herniæ in their early stages are reducible. Such a return may come about either spontaneously when the patient assumes the horizontal position, or it may not occur until pressure is applied in the form of taxis on the part of the patient or surgeon. When reduction is accomplished by taxis, the feeling of a solid body slipping away from the fingers is very apparent. If intestine form part of the contents of the sac, its reduction may moreover be accompanied by a very distinct gurgling sound or sensation. The contents of the sac met with in a reducible hernia may be varied, but bowel— and that usually small intestine or omentum of recent descent, are the most common viscera to be found within the sac." Eccles, pp. 18-19.
14. See Tillmanns, p. 180.
15. Hitzrot, p. 28.
16. Hudson, p. 142.
17. Warren, pp. 52 (a)-52 (d), Plate A.
18. *United States Armed Forces Medical Journal*, p. 191.
19. J. Johnson, p. 358.
20. J. Johnson, p. 409.
21. For instructions on taxis, or manually reducing a reducible inguinal hernia, see Deaver, p. 98.
22. See, e.g., Ranney, p. 347; Coats, p. 857; Love, pp. 233-244.
23. See Hare, *PM*, pp. 40-42.
24. See Tillmanns, p. 180.
25. See Keen and DeCosta, p. 27.
26. *Therapeutic Gazette*, p. 399.
27. Dorland, s.v. "hernia."
28. Dunglison, s.v. "Hernia."
29. Wyeth, p. 453. Note: Dr. Wyeth and I share a number of things in common, including a mutual reverence for our Southern and Confederate heritage, and I have cited material from his Confederate history in many of my own books on the War for Southern Independence.

30. Morris, p. 1397.
31. Morris, p. 1397.
32. Gray, p. 1049.
33. T. Bryant, p. 508.
34. Arnaud, p. 128.
35. Hoblyn, s.v. "Hernia."
36. Tillmanns, Vol. 3, p. 177.
37. Cheyne and Burghard, p. 417.
38. Stewart, p. 559.
39. Keen and DaCosta, p. 26.
40. Ranney, p. 344.
41. Warren, p. 27.
42. Cheyne and Burghard, p. 417; Warren, p. 28.
43. Edsall and Kent, p. 177.
44. Gour, pp. 260-261.
45. Gour, pp. 253-256.
46. Murray, pp. 13-16.
47. Harris, s.v. "hernia."
48. Marcy, *A Treatise on Hernia*, p. 1.
49. Ferguson, p. 9.
50. Dufour, pp. 38, 40-44.
51. Fröhner, pp. 185-186.
52. Fröhner, p. 186.
53. p. 313.
54. Keen and DaCosta, p. 59.
55. Keen and DaCosta, pp. 17-18.
56. *The Medical Council*, p. 119.
57. Marcy, *A Treatise on Hernia*, p. 33
58. Agnew, pp. 450-451.
59. Pierce, pp. 21-22. For a 1903-1911 list, see also *The Bellevue Hospital Nomenclature of Diseases and Conditions*, p. 43.
60. Foote, pp. 202-204.
61. De Garmo, p. 17.
62. Eccles, pp. 1-2.
63. *The Medical Council*, p. 119.
64. Dollar, p. 539.
65. Haubold, p. 2042.
66. Ashhurst, p. 1115.
67. Sultan, p. 51.
68. Sultan, p. 51.
69. *The Surgical Clinics of Chicago*, p. 21.
70. Fergusson, p. 632.
71. Stewart, p. 559.
72. *Special Bulletin*, pp. 8, 11.
73. Monro, p. 48.
74. Warwick, p. 1.
75. Eccles, pp. 4-5.
76. Eccles, p. 12.
77. Dufour, pp. 60-61.
78. De Garmo. p. 50.
79. Eccles, pp. 16-17.
80. Cheyne and Burghard, p. 417; Warren, p. 28.
81. Keen and DaCosta, p. 26.
82. Dowell, p. 21.

83. Goodhugh and Taylor, s.v. "Diseases."

84. Murray, pp. 1, 2.

85. Dr. Murray is using the word patent here in its medical sense: an "open and unobstructed vessel, duct, or aperture; or one that has failed to close." L.S.

86. Murray, pp. 11, 12.

87. Bilz, Vol. 1, pp. 621-622.

88. Arnaud, pp. 128-130.

89. Foote, pp. 204-205.

90. Agnew, pp. 451-452, 454, 455.

91. Gour, pp. 252-253, 256-257.

92. Warren, p. 25.

93. *The Medical Standard*, p. 14.

94. Ochsner and Percy, p. 391.

95. Goodwin, p. 393.

96. Hamilton, p. 725.

97. Lambert, Goldwater, and Lapp, p. 390.

98. Sultan, p. 52.

99. Lambert, Goldwater, and Lapp, p. 390.

100. *Illinois Medical Journal*, Vol. 27, 1915, p. 188. For more on this topic, see Taylor, pp. 330-332.

101. From Graser's *Handbook of Practical Surgery*, 1900, Vol. 20, p. 826.

102. See Hare, *PM*, pp. 40-42.

103. Stewart, p. 559.

104. Warren, p. 25.

105. Warren, pp. 26-28.

106. Tillmanns, pp. 179-180.

107. Ochsner, p. 231.

108. Edsall and Kent, p. 178.

109. Edsall and Kent, pp. 179-180.

110. Warren, p. 25.

111. Edsall and Kent, p. 180.

112. Keen and DaCosta, p. 27.

113. Keen and DaCosta, p. 17.

114. Keen and DaCosta, pp. 18-19.

115. Hayward, p. 6. In Medieval and ancient times numerous crude methods were employed to "cure" hernias, some so barbaric and outrageous they were later made illegal and banned. For some examples of these primitive practices, see Dowell, pp. 34-42.

116. Dufour, p. 16.

117. J. Johnson, p. 409.

118. Dufour, pp. 85-86.

119. Dufour, p. 16.

120. Arnaud, p. 157.

121. Agnew, p. 455.

122. Note: I do not recommend sit-ups for the self-healing of inguinal hernia. Speak to a qualified medical practitioner or fitness trainer to help you decide whether or not you should employ this particular exercise.

123. Note: Brief sessions of these same exercises would be considered anaerobic.

124. Bilz, Vol. 1, pp. 622-623.

125. For the source of Dr. Bilz's gymnastics program, see Shreiber, passim.

126. Bilz, Vol. 1, pp. 537-543.

127. Marcy, *A Treatise on Hernia*, p. 56.

128. Hayward, p. 4.

129. J. Johnson, p. 409.

130. See Hayward, p. 15; Dowell, pp. 43-44.

131. See Bilz, Vol. 1, p. 622.

132. See Lindlahr, p. 373.

133. See Lindlahr, pp. 156-162.

134. Bathing, and the general use of water for treating hernias of all kinds, was extremely common during the Victorian Period. See, e.g., Bowditch, p. 75; see Parrish, pp. 24, 68, 69, 73, 77, 78, 85,160, 176, 180, 196, 198, 204, 205, 244, 253, 262, 263, 286, 293, 294, 320.

135. Lindlahr, p. 373.

136. Gour, pp. 258-268.

137. J. Johnson, p. 409.

138. Lilienthal, s.v. "Hernia."

139. Dufour, p. 30.

140. Gour, p. 257.

141. For a complete and full discussion on the topic of the power of the mind, as well as the vital role the subconscious mind plays in both our health and our daily lives, see my book: *Jesus and the Law of Attraction*. Also see my books: *Christ is All and In All* and *The Bible and the Law of Attraction*.

142. See Hudson, p. 152.

143. De Garmo, p. 49.

144. *Illinois Medical Journal*, Vol. 1, 1899-1900, p. 246.

145. De Garmo. p. 50.

146. See Warren, pp. 23-24.

147. See Cheyne and Burghard, p. 417. They list "feeble [abdominal] muscles from faulty nutrition" as one of the leading causes of inguinal hernia.

148. Lindlahr, p. 371.

149. Warren, pp. 23-24.

150. For those interested, this form of eating is today called the Paleolithic diet. It has millions of followers—and for good reason.

151. Dufour, pp. 45-46.

152. See Sultan, p. 68.

153. Hayward, pp. 19-20.

154. Hayward, p. 20.

155. Shrady, p. 404.

156. Agnew, p. 457.

157. Shrady, p. 404.

158. Seabrook, *Jesus and the Law of Attraction*, pp. 47-49, 55-56.

159. Hudson, pp. 174-175.

160. Hudson, p. 154.

161. Philippians 4:8.

162. Lindlahr, p. 85.

163. See e.g., Mark 11:24. For more on this topic, see my book *Jesus and the Law of Attraction*.

164. Seabrook, *Jesus and the Law of Attraction*, p. 403.

165. Gage, p. 327. Note: From Ampère we derive the word "amp."

166. Seabrook, *Jesus and the Law of Attraction*, pp. 135-136.

167. Proverbs 23:7.

168. See Hudson, passim.

169. Hudson, p. 176.

170. See Hudson, pp. 199-204.

171. John 10:34.

172. See e.g., John 14:12.

173. Mark 9:23.

174. For more on the telepathic power of the subconscious mind, see the Introduction in my book *The Martian Anomalies*.

175. Luke 8:50.

176. See e.g., Dufour, pp. 69-70. Even shorter times have been reported. One health practitioner asserts that he cured a reducible hernia "in the course of a few weeks" using a decoction of oak tree bark. See J. Johnson, p. 409.

177. Bilz, Vol. 1, p. 561.

178. Bilz, Vol. 1, pp. 622-623.
179. Gour, p. 254.
180. Foote, p. 205.
181. Bilz, Vol. 1, p. 1044.
182. Dufour, p. 68.
183. Dufour, pp. 69-70.
184. Dufour, pp. 70-71.
185. Dufour, pp. 71-73.
186. Dufour, pp. 73-75.
187. Dufour, pp. 75-76.
188. Dufour, pp. 76-77.
189. Dufour, pp. 77-78.
190. Dufour, p. 79.
191. Dufour, pp. 79-80.
192. Dufour, pp. 80-81.
193. Dufour, pp. 81-83.
194. Dufour, pp. 83-84.
195. Dufour, pp. 84-85.
196. Dufour, pp. 85-86.
197. Dufour, pp. 86-87.
198. Foote, pp. 205-211.
199. Foote, pp. 377-378.
200. Foote, p. 374.

BIBLIOGRAPHY

And Suggested Reading

Abbot, Samuel L., and James C. White (eds.). *The Boston Medical and Surgical Journal.* Vol. 74. Boston, MA: David Clapp and Son, 1866.

Agnew, Hayes. *The Principles and Practice of Surgery: Being a Treatise on Surgical Diseases and Injuries.* 2 vols. Philadelphia, PA: J. B. Lippencott and Co., 1878.

Albright, Jacob D. *The General Practitioner as a Specialist.* Philadelphia, PA: self-published, 1904.

Annals of Surgery. Vol. 17, January to June 1893. Philadelphia, PA: University of Pennsylvania Press, 1893.

Annual Report of the Surgeon General, U.S. Navy, for the Fiscal Year 1926. Washington, D.C.: U.S. Dept of the Navy, Medicine and Surgery, 1926.

Annual Reports of the Navy Department for the Fiscal Year 1926. Washington, D.C.: U.S. Government Printing Office, 1927.

Arnaud, George. *A Dissertation on Hernias or Ruptures: In Two Parts.* London, UK: A. Millar, 1748.

Ashhurst, John (ed.). *The International Encyclopedia of Surgery.* 6 vols. New York: William Wood and Co., 1884.

Bedford, P. W. (ed.). *Pharmaceutical Record.* Vol. 9, January to December 1889. New York: The Pharmaceutical Record Co., 1890.

Billings, John S., and Robert Fletcher (eds.). *Index Medicus: Current Medical Literature of the World.* Vol. 19, May 1896 to April 1897. Boston, MA: self-published by the editors, 1897.

Bilz, Friedrich Eduard. *The Natural Method of Healing: A New and Complete Guide to Health.* 2 vols. Leipzig, Germany: self-published, 1898.

Boston With its Points of Interest. New York: Mercantile Illustrating Co., 1895.

Bowditch, Henry Ingersoll. *A Treatise on Diaphragmatic Hernia: Being an Account of a Case Observed at the Massachusetts General Hospital, Followed by a Numerical Analysis of All the Cases of This Affection, Found Recorded in the Writings of Medical Authors Between the Years 1610 and 1846.* Buffalo, NY: self-published, 1853.

Brickner, Walter M. (ed.). *American Journal of Surgery.* Vol. 33, 1919. New York: The Surgery Publishing Co., 1919.

Bryant, Joseph D. *Operative Surgery.* New York: D. Appleton and Co., 1908.

Bryant, Thomas. *A Manual for the Practice of Surgery.* Philadelphia, PA: Henry C. Lea's Son and Co., 1861.

Cheyne, W. Watson, and F. F. Burghard. 7 vols. *A Manual of Surgical Treatment.* Philadelphia, PA: Lea Brothers and Co., 1902.

Cornell University Medical Bulletin. Vol. 15, No. 1, July 1925. New York: Cornell University, 1925.

Covey, Alfred Dale. *The Secrets of Specialists: Incorporating Profitable Office Specialties.* Chicago, IL: Adams Publishing Co., 1916.

Deaver, John B. *Surgical Anatomy.* 3 vols. Philadelphia, PA: P. Blakiston's Son and Co., 1903.

De Garmo, William Burton. *Abdominal Hernia: Its Diagnosis and Treatment.* Philadelphia, PA: J. B. Lippencott Co., 1907.

Denison, Henry S., and George A. Moleen (eds.). *Colorado Medicine: A Medical Journal.* Vol. 6, January to December 1909. Denver, CO: The Merchants Publishing Co., 1909.

Dollar, John A. W. *Regional Veterinary Surgery and Operative Technique.* New York:

William R. Jenkins, 1912.

Dorland, W. A. Newman. *The American Illustrated Medical Dictionary*. Philadelphia, PA: W. B. Saunders and Co., 1916.

Dowell, Greensville. *A Treatise on Hernia: With a New Process for its Radical Cure, and Original Contributions to its Operative Surgery, and New Surgical Instruments*. Philadelphia, PA: D. G. Brinton, 1876.

Dufour, William. *A Treatise on the Radical Cure of Hernia or Rupture, by Intentional Means, With Cases, Most Unexceptionally Attested, Particularly by Overseers of Parishes and by Private Individuals, Effected Without any Surgical Operation, Pain, or Suspension of the Patient's Ordinary Avocations*. London, UK: C. Chapple, 1821.

Dunglison, Robley J. *A Dictionary of Medical Science*. Philadelphia, PA: Lea Brothers and Co., 1893.

Eccles, William McAdam. *Hernia: Its Etiology, Symptoms and Treatment*. New York: William Wood and Co., 1900.

Edsall, David L., and A. F. Stanley Kent (eds.). *The Journal of Industrial Hygiene*. Vol. 1, May 1919 to April 1920. Cambridge, MA: Macmillan Co., 1919-1920.

Edwards, Charles M. (ed.). *Virginia Medical Semi-Monthly*. Vol. 20, April 1915 to March 1916. Richmond, VA: Virginia Medical Society, 1916.

Eighth Biennial Report of the State Board of Control. October 1914 to September 1916. Olympia, WA: Washington State Government, 1916.

Eve, Paul F., and I. P. Garvin (eds.). *Southern Medical and Surgical Journal*. Vol. 1, 1845. Augusta, GA: P. C. Guieu, 1845.

Ferguson, Alexander Hugh. *The Technic of Modern Operations for Hernia*. Chicago, IL: Cleveland Press, 1908.

Fergusson, William. *A System of Practical Surgery*. London, UK: John Churchill and Sons, 1870.

Foote, Edward Bliss. *Medical Common Sense; Applied to the Causes, Prevention and Cure of Chronic Diseases and Unhappiness in Marriage*. New York: self-published, 1864.

Foster, Frank P. (ed.). *The New York Medical Journal*. Vol. 62, July to December 1895. New York: D. Appleton and Co., 1895.

Fröhner, Eugen. *Hand-Book of Veterinary Surgery and Obstetrics: Vol. 2, General Surgery*. Ithaca, NY: Taylor and Carpenter, 1906.

Furman, Bess. *A Profile of the United States Public Health Service, 1798-1948*. Washington, D.C.: U.S. Dept. of Health, Education, and Welfare, 1950.

Gage, Alfred Payson. *The Elements of Physics*. Boston, MA: Ginn and Co., 1898.

Goffe, J. Riddle (ed.). *The Medical News*. Vol. 71, June to December 1897. New York: Lea Brothers and Co., 1897.

Goldberg, Jane, with Jay Gutierrez. *The Hormesis Effect: The Miraculous Healing Power of Radioactive Stones*. Springhill, TN: Sea Raven Press, 2014.

Goodhugh, William, and William Cooke Taylor (eds.). *The Bible Cyclopedia*. London, UK: John W. Parker, 1841.

Goodwin, E. J. (ed.). *The Journal of the Missouri State Medical Association*. Vol. 22, January to December 1925. St. Louis, MO: Missouri State Medical Association, 1925.

Gour, Andrew Anastas. *The Therapeutics of Activity*. Chicago, IL: self-published, 1916.

Gray, Henry. *Anatomy, Descriptive and Surgical*. Philadelphia, PA: Lea Brothers and Co., 1901.

Hamilton, Frank Hastings. *The Principles and Practice of Surgery*. New York: William Wood and Co., 1876.

Hare, Hobart Amory (ed.). *Progressive Medicine*. Vol. 2, June 1902. Philadelphia,

PA: Lea and Febiger, 1902.

——. *The Therapeutic Gazette*. Vol. 41. Detroit, MI: E. G. Swift, 1917.

Harris, Chapin Aaron. *A Dictionary of Medical Terminology, Dental Surgery, and the Collateral Sciences*. Philadelphia, PA: Lindsay and Blakiston, 1855.

Hart, Ernest (ed.). *The British Medical Journal*. Vol. 1, January to June 1872. London, UK: Thomas Richards, 1872.

Hartelius, Truls Johan. *Home Gymnastics for the Preservation and Restoration of Health in Children and Young and Old People of Both Sexes*. Philadelphia, PA: J. B. Lippincott and Co., 1883.

Haubold, Herman A. *The Principles and Practice of Surgery*. New York: D. Appleton and Co., 1921.

Haupt, Barbara J., and Edmund Graves. *Detailed Diagnoses and Surgical Procedures for Patients Discharged from Short-Stay Hospitals*. Hyattsville, MD: U.S. Dept. of Health and Human Services, 1979.

Hayward, George. *Permanent Cure of Reducible Hernia*. Philadelphia, PA: self-published, 1852.

Heaton, George. *The Cure of Rupture: Reducible and Irreducible*. Boston, MA: H. O. Houghton and Co., 1877.

Hitzrot, James Morley (ed.). *Oxford Loose-Leaf Surgery*. London, UK: Oxford University Press, 1918.

Hoblyn, Richard Dennis. *A Dictionary of Terms Used in Medicine and the Collateral Sciences*. Philadelphia, PA: Henry C. Lea, 1865.

Hooper, Robert. *Lexicon Medicum; or Medical Dictionary*. London, UK: Longman, Orme and Co., 1839.

Howard, John. *Practical Observations of the Natural History and Cure of the Venereal Disease*. 2 vols. London, UK: self-published, 1806.

Hudson, Thomas Jay. *The Law of Psychic Phenomenon: A Working Hypothesis for the Systemic Study of Hypnotism, Spiritism, Mental Therapeutics, Etc.* 1893. Chicago, IL: A. C. McClurg and Co., 1905 ed.

Hyde, Walter Woodburn. *Olympic Victor Monuments and Greek Athletic Art*. Washington, D.C.: Carnegie Institute, 1921.

Illinois Medical Journal. Vol. 1, July 1899 to June 1900. Springfield, IL: Illinois State Journal Press, 1900.

——. Vol. 27, January to June 1915. Springfield, IL: Illinois State Journal Press, 1915.

International Journal of Surgery. Vol. 21, January to December 1908. New York: The International Journal of Surgery Co., 1908.

Johnson, James (ed.). *The Medico-Surgical Review, and Journal of Medical Science*. Vol. 3, 1822-1823. London, UK: Burgess and Hill, 1823.

Keen, William W., and John Chalmers DaCosta (eds.). *Surgery: Its Principles and Practice*. Vol. 4. 1908. Philadelphia, PA: W. B. Saunders and Co., 1914 ed.

Keen, William W., and J. William White (eds.). *An American Text-Book of Surgery for Practitioners and Students*. Philadelphia, PA: W. B. Saunders and Co., 1903.

Lambert, Alexander, S. S. Goldwater, and John A. Lapp (eds.). *Modern Medicine*. Vol.1, No. 1, 1919. Chicago, IL: Modern Medicine, 1919.

Lilienthal, Samuel. *Homeopathic Therapeutics*. New York: Boericke and Tafel, 1878.

Lindlahr, Henry. *Practice of Natural Therapeutics*. Chicago, IL: Lindlahr Publishing, 1919.

Love, Wilton. *Transactions of the Fifth Session of the Intercolonial Medical Congress of Australia, Held in Brisbane, Australia, September 1899*. Brisbane, Australia: Intercolonial Medical Congress of Australia, 1901.

Manley, Thomas H. *Hernia: Its Palliative and Radical Treatment in Adults, Children and Infants*. Philadelphia, PA: The Medical Press Co., 1893.

Marcy, Henry Orlando. *The Radical Cure of Hernia by the Antiseptic Use of the Carbolized Catgut Ligature*. Cambridge, MA: self-published, 1879.

——. *A Treatise on Hernia: The Radical Cure by the Use of the Buried Antiseptic Animal Suture*. Detroit, MI: George C. Davis, 1889.

McCormack, Arthur T. (ed.). *Kentucky Medical Journal*. Vol. 20, January to December 1922. Bowling Green, KY: Kentucky State Medical Association, 1922.

McCurdy, James H. *A Bibliography of Physical Training*. Springfield, MA: Physical Directors' Society of the Young Men's Christian Association of North America, 1905.

McMichael, Arkell Robert. *A Compendium of Materia Medica, Therapeutics and Repertory of the Digestive System*. Philadelphia, PA: Boericke and Tafel, 1892.

Monro, Alexander. *Observations on Crural Hernia: To Which is Prefixed a General Account of the Other Varieties of Hernia*. Edinburgh, Scotland: W. Laing, 1803.

Morris, Henry. *Morris' Human Anatomy: A Complete Systematic Treatise*. Philadelphia, PA: P. Blakiston's Son and Co., 1935.

Moses, Adolph (ed.). *The National Corporation Register*. Vol. 6, March 1893 to September 1893. Chicago, IL: The United States Corporation Bureau, 1893.

Murray, Robert William. *Hernia: Its Cause and Treatment*. London, UK: J and A Churchill, 1908.

New England Medical Monthly. Vol. 19, No. 1, January 1900. Boston, MA: Boston Medical Library, 1900.

New York State Journal of Medicine. Vol. 23, No. 1, May 22, 1923. New York: The Medical Society of the State of New York, 1923.

Ochsner, Albert John, and Nelson M. Percy (eds.). *A New Clinical Surgery*. Chicago, IL: Cleveland Press, 1912.

Ochsner, Albert John. (ed.). *Surgical Diagnosis and Treatment*. Philadelphia, PA: Lea and Febiger, 1921.

Ohmann-Dumesnil, A. H. (ed.). *The St. Louis Medical and Surgical Journal*. Vol. 86, January to June 1904. St. Louis, MO: self-published, 1904.

O'Leary, James. *A History of the Bible: Its Origin, Object, and Structure*. New York: P. J. Kennedy, 1898.

Pacific Medical Journal. Vol. 36, No. 1, January to December 1893. San Francisco, CA: no publisher, 1893.

Parrish, Joseph. *Practical Observations on Strangulated Hernia, and Some of the Diseases of the Urinary Organs*. Philadelphia, PA: Key and Biddle, 1836.

Pierce, C. C. (ed.). *Nomenclature of Diseases and Conditions*. Washington, D.C.: U.S. Treasury Dept. and U.S. Public Health Service, 1921.

Pokras, Robert, and Vicki Hufnagel. *Vital and Health Statistics: Data From the National Health Survey*. Series 13, No. 92. Washington, D.C.: Public Health Service, 1987.

Punton, John (ed.). *The Kansas City Medical-Lancet*. Vol. 22, January to December 1901. Kansas City, MO: self-published, 1901.

Quarterly Cumulative Index to Current Medical Literature. Vol. 5, January to December 1920. Chicago, IL: American Medical Association, 1921.

Ranking, W. H., and C. B. Radcliffe (eds.). *American Medical Times*. Vol. 1, No. 2, July 14, 1860. New York: New York Journal of Medicine, 1860.

Ranney, Ambrose L. *A Practical Treatise on Surgical Diagnosis*. New York: William Wood and Co., 1881.

Rich, Burdett A., and M. Blair Wailes (eds.). *American Law Reports Annotated*. Vol. 20. Rochester, NY: The Lawyers Co-operative Publishing Co., 1922.

Sajous, Charles E. *Sajous's Analytical Cyclopedia of Practical Medicine*. Philadelphia, PA: F. A. Davis Co., 1904.

Schreber, Daniel Gottlieb Moritz. *Illustrated Medical Indoor Gymnastics*. London, UK: Williams, 1856.

Seabrook, Lochlainn. *Jesus and the Law of Attraction: The Bible-Based Guide to Creating Perfect Health, Wealth, and Happiness Following Christ's Simple Formula*. Spring Hill, TN: Sea Raven Press, 2013.

——. *The Bible and the Law of Attraction: 99 Teachings of Jesus, the Apostles, and the Prophets*. 2013. Spring Hill, TN: Sea Raven Press, 2020 ed.

——. *Christ is All and in All: Rediscovering Your Divine Nature and the Kingdom Within*. 2014. Spring Hill, TN: Sea Raven Press, 2020 ed.

——. *Seabrook's Bible Dictionary of Traditional and Mystical Christian Doctrines*. Spring Hill, TN: Sea Raven Press, 2016.

——. *Vintage Southern Cookbook: 2,000 Delicious Dishes From Dixie*. Spring Hill, TN: Sea Raven Press, 2021.

——. *The Martian Anomalies: A Photographic Search for Intelligent Life on Mars*. Spring Hill, TN: Sea Raven Press, 2022.

——. *Vitamin D: The Miracle Treatment for Nearly Every Disease and Health Issue*. Cody, WY: Sea Raven Press, 2024.

Shattuck, George B. (ed.). *The Boston Medical and Surgical Journal*. Vol. 151, July to December 1904. Boston, MA: The Old Corner Book Store, 1904.

Shrady, George F. (ed.). *The Medical Record*. Vol. 29, December 1885 to June 1886. New York: William Wood and Co., 1886.

Special Bulletin: Labor and Industry. No. 6. Harrisburg, PA: Pennsylvania Dept. of Labor and Industry, 1925.

Stengel, Alfred. *A Text-Book of Pathology*. Philadelphia, PA: W. B. Saunders and Co., 1901.

Stewart, Francis T. *A Manual of Surgery for Students and Physicians*. Philadelphia, PA: P. Blakiston's Son and Co., 1915.

Story, John B. (ed.). *Transactions of the Royal Academy of Medicine in Ireland*. Vol. 18. Dublin, Ireland: Fannin and Co., 1899.

Sultan, Georg. *Atlas and Epitome of Abdominal Hernias*. Philadelphia, PA: W. B. Saunders and Co., 1892.

Taylor, Holman. *Texas State Journal of Medicine*. Vol. 8, May 1912 to April 1913. Fort Worth, TX: The Exline-Reimers Co., 1913.

The Bellevue Hospital Nomenclature of Diseases and Conditions. New York: Bellevue Board of Trustees, 1911.

The British and Foreign Medico-Surgical Review. Vol. 37, January to April 1866. London, UK: John Churchill and Sons, 1866.

The Bulletin of the Battle Creek Sanitarium and Hospital Clinic. Vol. 21, No. 1, January 1926. Battle Creek, MI: Medical Faculty of the Battle Creek Sanitarium, 1926.

The Chicago Medical Recorder. Vol. 2, September 1891 to February 1892. Chicago, IL: W. T. Keener, 1892.

The Johns Hopkins Hospital Bulletin. Vol. 4. Baltimore, MD: The Press of the Friedenwald Co., 1893.

The Journal of the American Medical Society. Vol. 36, No. 14, April 1901. Chicago, IL: American Medical Society, 1901.

The Lancet. Vol. 1, January to June 1862. London, UK: George Fall, 1862.

The Medical Council. Vol. 25, No. 1., January to December 1920. Philadelphia, PA: The Medical Council Co., 1920.

The Medical Herald. Vol. 35, No. 1, January 1916. Kansas City, MO: Medical Society of the Missouri Valley, 1916.

The Medical Standard. Vol. 18, January to December 1896. Chicago, IL: G. P. Engelhard and Co., 1896.

The Surgical Clinics of Chicago. Vol. 1. Philadelphia, PA: W. B. Saunders and Co., 1917.

Tillmanns, Hermann. *A Text-Book of Surgery*. New York: D. Appleton and Co., 1898.

Transactions of the American Association of Obstetricians and Gynecologists. Vol. 26, for the year 1913. York, PA: The Maple Press, 1914.

Transactions of the Medical Society of the State of New York for the Year 1902. Albany, NY: The Medical Society of the State of New York, 1902.

Transactions of the Philadelphia Academy of Surgery. Vol. 18, January 1915 to December 1915. Philadelphia, PA: self-published, 1916.

Transactions of the Seventh Session of the Australian Medical Congress, Held at Adelaide, September 1905. Adelaide, South Australia: self-published, 1907.

Transactions of the Thirty-Third Annual Meeting of the Mississippi Valley Medical Association, Held in Columbus, Ohio, October 8-10, 1907. Cincinnati, OH: The Lancet-Clinic, 1908.

United States Armed Forces Medical Journal. Vol. 2, No. 1, January 1960. Washington, D.C.: U.S. Dept. of Defense, 1960.

Warren, Joseph H. *A Practical Treatise on Hernia*. London, UK: Sampson Low, Marston, Searle, and Rivington, 1880.

Warwick, Bruce Lester. *A Study of Hernia in Swine*. Madison, WI: Agricultural Experiment Station of the University of Wisconsin and U.S. Dept. of Agriculture Co-operating, 1926.

Wiseman, Richard. *Eight Surgical Treatises*. London, UK: 1719.

Wyeth, John Allan. *Surgery*. New York: Marion Sims Wyeth and Co., 1908.

Ziegler, Ernst. *A Text-Book of Pathological Anatomy and Pathogenesis*. New York: William Wood and Co., 1884.

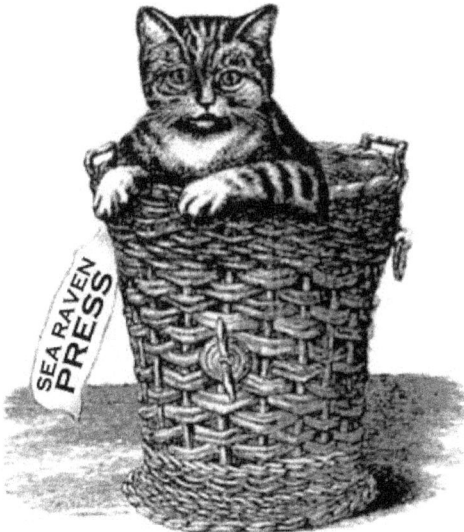

INDEX

SEA RAVEN PRESS

was founded for the express purpose of publishing and circulating such books as are calculated to store the mind with useful knowledge. We therefore publish only books of a high moral tone and tendency—such works as will be welcomed in every home and at every fireside as valuable family treasures.

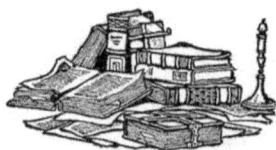

L. SEABROOK

✷ "I love Lochlainn Seabrook's style and approach. It's not the 'norm.' What a miracle his books are. . . . He is a literal life changing author! Amazing books!" — KEITH PARISH

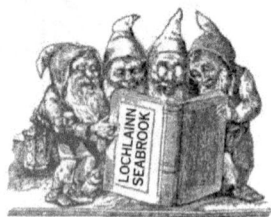

✷ "I adore Mr. Seabrook's style and I love his books. I love an author that does proper research, and still finds a way to engage the reader. Mr. Seabrook does an admirable job of both." — DONALD CAUL

✷ "Lochlainn Seabrook's books are much more well researched and authoritative than those eminently celebrated as being the authorities on the subjects he writes on. You can always trust to find the truth in his writings. . . . He does not rewrite history, but instead shows it as it is." — GARY STIER

✷ "I love all of Colonel Seabrook's books. They are informative and enlightening, and his warm Southern hospitality writing style makes you feel right at home." — KEITH CRAVEN

✷ "Lochlainn Seabrook's work is an absolute treasure of scholarship and historic scope." — MARK WAYNE CUNNINGHAM

✷ "Mr. Seabrook's command of . . . history is breathtaking. . . . He deserves great renown—check out his books!" — MARGARET SIMMONS

✷ "I love Seabrook's writings. LOVE!!! . . . So grateful to know the truth! Keep writing Lochlainn!!!" — REBECCA DALRYMPLE

✷ "Lochlainn Seabrook . . . [has] probably [written] the best book on mental science in existence by a living author. Along with Thomas Troward, Emmet Fox, and Jack Addington, Mr. Seabrook is one of the top four mental science authors of all time, since biblical times." - IAN BARTON STEWART

✷ "Glad I discovered Mr. Seabrook! . . . He writes eye opening books! Unbelievable the facts he unearths - and he backs it all up with truth, notes, footnotes, and bibliography! . . . He always amazes me! His books always see the whole picture. His timelines and bibliographies are incredible. He always provides carefully reasoned arguments! He's the best. To me I think he's better than the late great Shelby Foote! America needs more like Lochlainn Seabrook. I can't wait to own all of his books on the war someday. Everyone who wants the Truth, who seeks the Truth and wants the full story, should read his books." — JOHN BULL BADER

✷ "I love all of Colonel Seabrook's books!" — DEBBIE SIDLE

✷ "Lochlainn Seabrook is well educated and versed in what he writes and I'm impressed with the delivery." — THOMAS L. WHITE

✷ "Thank you Lochlainn Seabrook for your wonderful books! You are the real deal! You are an amazing author and I love your books!!" — SOPHIA MEOW CELLIST

✷ "I really enjoy Mr. Seabrook's books! His knowledge is beyond belief!" — SANDRA FISH

✷ "Love Lochlainn Seabrook. Awesome!!" — ROBIN HENDERSON ARISTIDES

✷ "Kudos to Lochlainn Seabrook who is a very good and informative professional truthful historian. We need more like him!" — AMY VACHON

MEET THE AUTHOR

"Bestselling author, award-winning historian, and esteemed nature writer Lochlainn Seabrook straddles multiple genres with ease, seamlessly weaving together history, science, politics, philosophy, and spirituality with the authority of a scholar and the flair of a storyteller." — SEA RAVEN PRESS

AMERICAN POLYMATH **LOCHLAINN SEABROOK** is a bestselling author, award-winning historian, and world acclaimed artist. A descendant of the families of Alexander Hamilton Stephens, John Singleton Mosby, Edmund Winchester Rucker, and William Giles Harding, the neo-Victorian scholar is a 7th generation Kentuckian, and one of the most prolific and widely read traditional writers in the world today. Known by literary critics as the "new Shelby Foote," the "American Robert Graves," the "Southern Joseph Campbell," and the "Rocky Mountain Richard Jefferies," and by his fans as the "the best author ever," he is a recipient of the United Daughters of the Confederacy's prestigious Jefferson Davis Historical Gold Medal, and is considered the foremost Southern interpreter of American Civil War history—or what he refers to as the War for the Constitution (1861-1865).

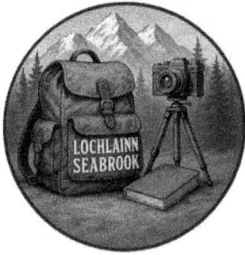

A lifelong litterateur, the Sons of Confederate Veterans member has authored and edited books ranging in topics from ancient and modern history, politics, science, comparative religion, diet and nutrition, spirituality, astronomy, entertainment, military, biography, mysticism, anthropology, cryptozoology, photography, and Bible studies, to natural history, technology, paleography, music, humor, gastronomy, etymology, paleontology, onomastics, mysteries, alternative health and fitness, wildlife, alternate history, comparative mythology, genealogy, Christian history, and the paranormal; books that his readers describe as "game changers," "transformative," and "life altering."

One of America's most popular living historians, nature writers, and Transcendentalists, he is a 17th generation Southerner of Appalachian heritage who descends from dozens of patriotic Revolutionary War soldiers and Confederate soldiers from Kentucky, Tennessee, North Carolina, and Virginia. Also a history, wildlife, and nature preservationist, the well-respected scrivener began life as a child prodigy, later maturing into an archetypal Renaissance Man.

Besides being cofounder and co-CEO of Sea Raven Press, an accomplished writer, author, historian, biographer, lexicographer, encyclopedist, neologist, publisher, editor, poet, creative, onomastician, etymologist, and Bible authority, the influential prosateur is also a Kentucky Colonel, eagle scout, entrepreneur, businessman, composer, screenwriter, nature, wildlife, and landscape photographer, videographer, and filmmaker, artist, artisan, painter, watercolorist, sculptor, ceramic artist, visual artist, sketch artist, pen and ink artist, graphic artist, graphic designer, book designer, book formatter, editorial designer, book cover designer, publishing designer, Web designer, poster artist, digital artist, cartoonist, content creator, inventor, aquarist, genealogist, ufologist, jewelry designer, jewelry maker, former history museum docent, teacher's assistant, and a former Red Cross certified lifeguard, ranch hand, zookeeper, and wrangler. A contemporary songwriter (of some 3,000 songs in a dozen genres), he is also a pianist, organist, drummer, bass player, rhythm guitarist, rhythm mandolinist, percussionist, electronic musician, synthesist, clavichordist, harpsichordist, classical composer, jingle composer, film composer (currently his musical work has been featured in 11 movies), lyricist, band leader, multi-instrument musician, lead vocalist, backup vocalist, session player, music producer, and recording studio mixing engineer, who has worked and performed with some of Nashville's top musicians and singers.

Currently Seabrook is the multi-genre author and editor of over 100 adult and children's books (totaling some 30,000 pages and 15,000,000 words) in over 100 categories, books that have earned him accolades from around the globe. His works, which have sold on every continent except Antarctica, have introduced hundreds of thousands to vital facts that have been left out of our mainstream books. He has been endorsed internationally by leading experts, museum curators, award-winning historians, chart-topping authors, celebrities, filmmakers, noted scientists, well regarded educators, TV show hosts and producers, renowned military artists, venerable heritage organizations, and distinguished academicians of all races, creeds, and colors.

He currently holds two interesting world records: He is the author of the most books on American military officer Nathan Bedford Forrest (12 in total), and he was the first to publicize and describe the 19th-Century platform reversal of America's two main political parties, namely that Civil War era Democrats (primarily in the South—the Confederacy) were Conservatives, while Civil War era Republicans (primarily in the North—the Union) were Liberals.

Of northern, western, and central European ancestry, he is the 6th great-grandson of the Earl of Oxford and a descendant of European royalty through his Kentucky father and West Virginia mother. A proud descendant of Appalachian coal miners, trainmen, mountain folk, and wilderness pioneers, his modern day cousins include: Johnny Cash, Elvis Presley, Lisa Marie Presley, Billy Ray and Miley Cyrus, Patty Loveless, Tim McGraw, Lee Ann Womack, Dolly Parton, Pat Boone, Naomi, Wynonna, and Ashley Judd, Ricky Skaggs, the Sunshine Sisters, Martha Carson, Chet Atkins, Patrick J. Buchanan, Cindy Crawford, Bertram Thomas Combs (Kentucky's 50th governor), Edith Bolling (second wife of President Woodrow Wilson), Andy Griffith, Riley Keough, George C. Scott, Robert Duvall, Reese Witherspoon, Lee Marvin, Rebecca Gayheart, and Tom Cruise.

A constitutionalist, avid outdoorsman, wilderness conservationist, and gun rights advocate, Seabrook is the author of the international blockbuster, *Everything You Were Taught About the Civil War is Wrong, Ask a Southerner!* He lives with his wife and family in the magnificent Rocky Mountains, heart of the American West, where you will find him writing, hiking, and filming.

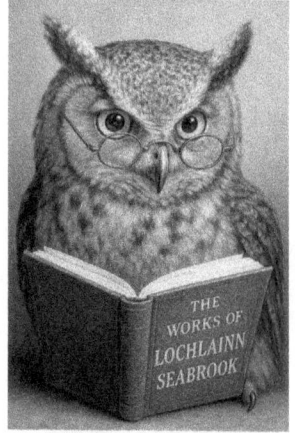

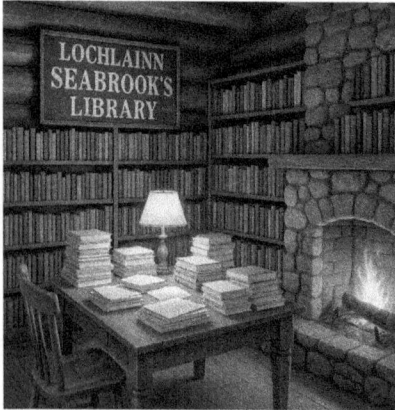

FOR MORE INFORMATION ON MR. SEABROOK VISIT

LOCHLAINNSEABROOK.COM

If you enjoyed this book you will be interested in Col. Seabrook's popular related title:

☛ VITAMIN D: THE MIRACLE TREATMENT FOR NEARLY EVERY DISEASE & HEALTH ISSUE

Available from Sea Raven Press and wherever fine books are sold

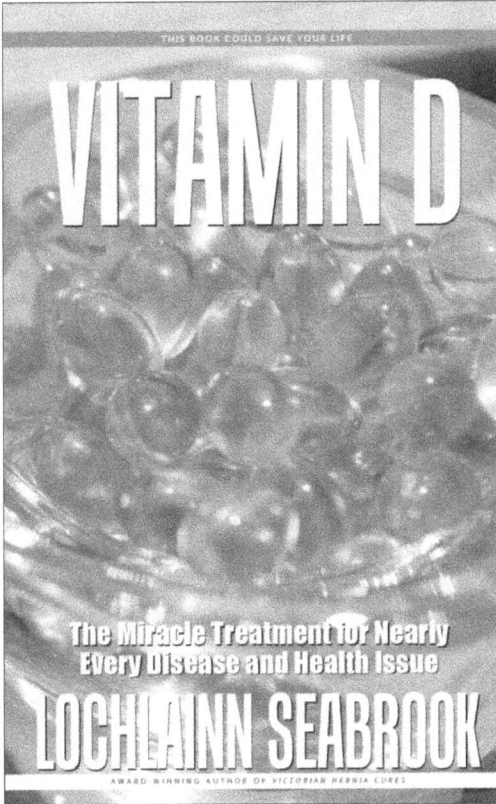

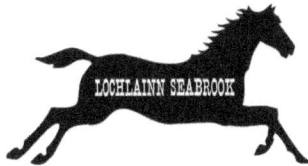

SeaRavenPress.com